"I love this book! Suza Francina breaks new ground in *Yo~* *Menopause.* She sheds light on a subject that has long is a gift to women at this time in their lives. I lov Sisterhood—to women everywhere. I wish I'd had this

author and host of the groundbreaking ~~..., ~oga and You

"Author and yoga teacher Suza Francina presents a wide range of useful and important information about menopause, and at the same time draws the reader in with very personal and fascinating stories from real women as they go through 'the change.' I couldn't put it down."

—Judith Hanson Lasater, Ph.D.
physical therapist and yoga teacher, author of *Relax and Renew: Restful Yoga for Stressful Times* and *Living Your Yoga: Finding the Spiritual in Every Day Life*

"Suza Francina gives inspirational support for women going through menopause. She encourages women to find and nurture their inner wisdom. Incorporating yoga, up-to-date information and heartfelt stories, this is a 'must-read' for all women who want to live their lives fully. I drank every word of this book into my being!"

—Elise Browning Miller, M.A.
senior certified Iyengar yoga teacher,
coauthor, *Life Is a Stretch: Easy Yoga, Anytime, Anywhere*

"In my twenty-five years of practice I've seen hundreds of women healed by herbal and natural therapies, and now *Yoga and the Wisdom of Menopause* is an essential part of my efforts to help more women have a graceful change. Epona, the goddess of horses, will be deeply grateful for all the canceled Premarin prescriptions once this book hits the stands!"

—Amanda McQuade Crawford, Dip. Phyto, MNIMH
founder, The American Herbalists Guild,
author, *The Herbal Menopause Book* and *Herbal Remedies for Women*

"What separates this book from the multitude of books on yoga these days, are the personal stories. They invite women to come together in mutual healing, strength and commitment to a life lived fully on all levels. Many thanks to Suza Francina for her work."

—Gaye Abbott, R.Y.T.
integrative yoga therapist, women's retreat leader

"Developing a yoga practice with Suza's guidance will make a world of difference in the quality of your midlife adventure. She is a remarkable and compassionate teacher."

—Rita Rivest
director of Sage Hill Retreat for Women

"*Yoga and the Wisdom of Menopause* is an amazing gift! It is so rich, well researched, sensible and insightful. I hope women everywhere read it. This book will be the bible for women everywhere moving into their power years."

—Cheryl Gilman
author, *Doing Work You Love: Discovering Your Purpose, Realizing Your Dreams*

"Here's a book I feel is destined to become a classic in its field. Suza Francina is an intelligent writer, with a keen understanding of both the many health issues surrounding menopause and the ways in which the yoga asanas can be used to treat them. She's put together just the right mix of concrete information and personal testimony, which gives her readers both a practical course of self-help study and supportive companionship along the way."

—Richard Rosen
deputy director, Yoga Research and Education Center
contributing editor, *Yoga Journal*
author, *The Yoga of Breath: A Step-by-Step Guide to Pranayama*

"A wonderfully wise and empowering book by a remarkable woman who's a real rarity—not only is she a pioneering yoga teacher, but she is also a compassionate and courageous politician, who served as Mayor of Ojai, California!"

—Corinne McLaughlin
co-founder of the Center for Visionary Leadership
coauthor of *Spiritual Politics: Changing the World from the Inside Out*

"I savored it, and at times absolutely devoured it, thoroughly enjoying its wisdom and verve. Rock on, wise women of yoga!"

—Leza Lowitz
author, *Yoga Poems: Lines to Unfold By*

"What impressed me about this book was the confidence it gave to the reader to trust in the body's innate ability to heal itself with a consistent and mindful yoga practice. Suza's book makes you realize that yoga is one of the best gifts we can give to ourselves."

—Susan Rosen, RYT
Yoga teacher, breast cancer survivor
producer of the video *Yoga and the Gentle Art of Healing:
A Journey of Recovery After Breast Cancer*

"It's surprising that there is so little out there that explores the benefits that yoga can have for women at this time in their lives. Francina's book is not only sorely needed, it's long overdue."

—Janiss Garza
editor, *Allspiritfitness.com*

YOGA AND THE WISDOM OF MENOPAUSE

A Guide to Physical, Emotional and Spiritual Health at Midlife and Beyond

SUZA FRANCINA

Health Communications, Inc.
Deerfield Beach, Florida

www.bcibooks.com

We would like to acknowledge the publishers and individuals below for permission to reprint the following material:

Photographs of Linda DiCarlo by Scott Wagers

Photographs of Suza Francina, Malchia Olshan, Catherine Meek by Ruth Miller, Nature's Studio Photography, Ojai, California

Photograph of Judith Hanson Lasater by Seth Affoumado

Photographs of Carin Seebold by Paul Bowden

Photographs of Maggie Mellor by Christopher Mellor

Photograph of Denise Lampron by Loretta Warner

Photograph of Susan Winter Ward by David Watersun

Photographs of Ingrid Boulting by Douglas Dubler

Photograph of Julie Lawrence by Ancil Nance

Photographs of Ana Forrest by Nils Vidsrand Photography, Los Angeles

Photographs of Virginia Lee by Susan Rogers-Sasher

Photograph of Gaye Abbott and Leza Lowitz by Dawn M. Justice

Quotes from *Relax & Renew: Restful Yoga for Stressful Times,* by Judith Lasater, Ph.D., P.T. ©1995 by Judith Lasater, Ph.D., P.T. Reprinted with permission of Rodmell Press, Berkeley, CA.

Photograph of Suza Francina, page xvi, Timothy Teague Photography

Photograph of Suza Francina, page 57, Paul Del Signore Photography

Photograph of Diana Rose Hartmann, page 77, by Anna Hartmann

Library of Congress Cataloging-in-Publication Data

Francina, Suza
   Yoga and the wisdom of menopause : a guide to physical, emotional, and spiritual health at midlife and beyond / Suza Francina.
      p.   cm.
   ISBN 0-7573-0065-0
      1. Menopause—Alternative treatment.   2. Yoga—Health aspects.   3. Middle aged women—Health and hygiene.   I. Title.

RG186.F73 2003
618.1'7506—dc21   2003044974

©2003 Suza Francina
ISBN 0-7573-0065-0

Publisher: Health Communications, Inc.
             3201 S.W. 15th Street
             Deerfield Beach, Florida 33442-8190

R-07-03

Cover design by Andrea Perrine Brower
Inside book design by Lawna Patterson Oldfield
Cover photo of Linda DiCarlo by Scott Wagers

To the Yoga Sisterhood

Contents

Author's Note: Crossing the Menopausal Bridge xi

Introduction: Welcome to Yoga and the Wisdom of Menopause xv

Why I Am Writing This Book xix

How This Book Can Help You xxiii

Judith Hanson Lasater: Menopause Was What Happened to

Older Women—Not Me xxviii

1. The Yoga of Menopause: Alternatives to Hormone Therapy 1

Yoga's Unique Benefits During the Menopausal Years 2

What Is Menopause? 3

Hormones 101 5

A Word on Weight Gain During Menopause 8

Key Poses to Help Balance Your Hormones 10

Carin Seebold: I Did Not Want to Take Hormone Replacement Therapy . . . 11

Gretchen Newmark: I Found I Needed Hormones! 17

Ingrid Boulting: Smooth Transition Due to Yoga and Diet 20

2. Yoga and the Endocrine System 23

The Endocrine Glands 25

Yoga, Menopause and Thyroid Function 27

The Adrenal Glands: Mood Swings and Fatigue 27

The Adrenal Hormones and Tolerating Stress 29

Yoga for Adrenal Health 31

Yoga's Great Rejuvenators—Essential Poses for Crossing the
　　Menopausal Bridge 33
Benefits of Yoga on the Endocrine System. 37
Key Poses for Adrenal Exhaustion and Fatigue 41
Julie Lawrence: First Find Rest 42
Linda DiCarlo: Compared to My Younger Years, I Now Practice
　　with More Intelligence and Wisdom 46
Interview with Patricia Walden: This Is Not the Time to Take
　　On More Things 50

3. Yoga for Pelvic Health During Perimenopause and Menopause . . . 57
Yoga's Healing Effect on the Uterus and Ovaries. 58
Yoga for Frequent or Irregular Bleeding 59
Cautions About Upside-Down (Inverted) Poses When Bleeding. 62
Upside-Down Poses After the Menstrual Period. 65
Yoga to Alleviate Pelvic Congestion, Pelvic Pain and Cramps 67
Menstrual Problems and Nutritional Remedies 68
Key Poses for Pelvic Health 71
Diana Rose Hartmann: Tossed Over the Bridge into Menopause 73

4. The Power of Hot Flashes 79
Alternative Theories on Hot Flashes 81
Hot Flashes May Be Healthy. 82
Cooling Yoga Poses for Hot Flashes, Day/Night Sweats and Other
Menopausal Symptoms 83
Key Poses to Ease Hot Flashes 91
Interview with Susan Winter Ward: Embracing Menopause:
　　A Path to Peace and Power. 92

5. Yoga Builds Healthy Bones 97
Your Skeleton: The Body's Calcium Bank Account 100
Bone Density and Osteoporosis 101
Building Healthy Bones Without Drugs. 102
Why Yoga Is a Superior Form of Weight-Bearing Exercise 105

Yoga and Preventing Height Loss 109
Safe Yoga for Osteoporosis 111
Key Poses for Strong Bones 115
Gaye Abbott: Deep Discoveries About Healing from Osteoporosis. 116
Elizabeth Memel: Yoga Strengthened My Bones After
    Chemotherapy for Breast Cancer 120

6. Yoga for Coping with Cancer 125
The Current Status of Cancer Research and Treatment. 126
Practicing Yoga to Reduce Breast Cancer Risk. 127
Yoga for Breast Health 129
Yoga Poses for Women in Breast Cancer Treatment. 131
Key Poses for a Healthy Immune System 137
Catherine Meek: Ahhh, Yoga—
    It Kept Me Sane and Made Me Whole Again. 138
Maggie Mellor: My Journey Through Breast Cancer—
    How Yoga Helped Me 141

7. Yoga for a Woman's Heart 145
A Woman's Heart: Where Body, Mind and Spirit Converge 146
Differences Between Women and Men in Heart Disease 147
Taking Your Emotions to Heart 153
Stress, Yoga and the Heart 154
Posture Also Affects the Health of Your Heart 157
Key Poses for Heart Health and High Blood Pressure 162
Virginia Lee: A Time of Moving into the Wisdom of Cronehood 163
Denise Lamprom: Menopause as a Spiritual Gateway 169

8. Yoga and the Wisdom of Menopause Practice Guide 177
Perimenopause Yoga Practice Guidelines. 180
Yoga Props—An Investment in Your Health. 181

How the Poses in This Guide Are Organized 184

Section I: Essential Restorative Yoga Poses for Crossing
  the Menopausal Bridge. 185

Section II: Standing Forward Bends and
  Supported Downward-Facing Dog Pose 200

Section III: Supported Standing Poses 206

Section IV: Important Seated and Lying Down Poses During Menopause. . 216

Section V: Poses Using Wall Ropes and Inversion Slings 223

Lying Back Over a Backbender 229

Section VI: Key Poses to Learn Under the Guidance of a Teacher 230

Ana Forrest: Strength and Spirit 238

Resources 243
Bibliography and References 253
Index of Poses 267
About the Author 269

Author's Note

Crossing the Menopausal Bridge

Those of us walking across the menopausal bridge today owe a great debt to the pioneering women who lifted menopause out of the dark ages and brought it into the light of day. These women dispelled myths, lifted the veil of ignorance and elevated menopause from a hormone deficiency disease to a new and higher stage in life: the Wise Woman stage.

One of these pioneers was Gail Sheehy. During the course of writing this book, I had the opportunity to consider the deeper meaning of the title of her pathbreaking book, *The Silent Passage*.

Her title carries echoes of another revolutionary work, Rachel Carson's *Silent Spring*. Rachel Carson helped give birth to the environmental movement in the early 1960s when she wrote about the pollution of our air and water. Her book foresaw a dreadful day when the spring would be silent—when pollution would destroy the reproductive cycles of the birds, and they would no longer sing their songs.

The Silent Passage echoes that notion. It implies that in menopause, the clear and vibrant voice of women had been stilled—we had been silenced. Then, we demanded that our collective voices be heard and listened to!

During the passage of adolescence, our voices are exuberant. We celebrate that change. We flaunt it! We are out there on MTV with it. But who is the goddess of menopause?

To me, that individual is Christiane Northrup, M.D., author of *The Wisdom of Menopause*. We can thank Dr. Northrup, and all the other pioneering women before her, for helping us to celebrate this liberating, crowning, glorious stage of life.

Long before Dr. Northrup appeared on the scene, a trail of other physicians, both men and women, ruffled the feathers of the medical establishment and urged women to take control of their own health and choose a doctor who listens and provides proper respect and care. We can thank medical heretics like Robert S. Mendelsohn, M.D., who, in the early 1980s, was among the first physicians to sound the alarm on the medicalization of menopause. His book, *Male Practice: How Doctors Manipulate Women,* warned women about the adverse effects of Premarin, a substance derived from the urine of pregnant mares (*Pre*gnant *mar*e urine—see the Resources section for more information on this utterly inhumane practice). He also alerted them to the risks of the most indiscriminately recommended surgical procedures—the hysterectomy and radical mastectomy. He described the hazards associated with the prolonged use of conjugated estrogens, including uterine cancer, blood clots, liver tumors and high blood pressure. His comments proved remarkably prophetic.

Often we don't realize what unconscious ideas we have about a subject until we are introduced to a whole new way of thinking about it. Such was the case in the early 1990s when one of my students further revolutionized my thinking regarding menopause. She brought to one of my yoga classes a video whose title boldly declared, *Celebrate the Transition! Menopause: Dispelling the Myths, Telling the Truths, Exploring the Possibilities.* Among the women featured were Jesse Hanley, M.D., one of the early women doctors to advocate natural approaches to restoring hormone balance, and herbalist and naturopathic physician Farida Sharan, N.D., author of *Creative Menopause,* who further illuminated my understanding of women's health and spirituality.

There is not enough space to thank all the Wise Woman healers whose combined energies are bringing about a new paradigm in women's health, but I must give special thanks to Susun S. Weed, one of the mothers of herbal medicine in our country. Her recently revised and updated classic, *Menopausal Years: The Wise Woman Way,* brings together all the dimensions of menopause.

I applaud the way she has brought ancient wisdom into our modern era.

The sources for the yoga and menopause information in this book are from yoga master B.K.S. Iyengar and his daughter Geeta S. Iyengar, an expert on yoga for women and author of *Yoga: A Gem for Women.* As I adjusted my own practice during menopause, I grew to appreciate the wisdom of her simple advice to women going through the change: "First find rest. . . . If the body wants to slow down, you have to allow it to slow down for a while."

I realize now that many of my early teachers began yoga during their own menopause. My very first teacher, a woman in her early fifties, told me that she started yoga because she was looking for "exercise without exhaustion." Another teacher, Felicity Green, frequently told her menopausal students, "Your body is going through a change and you have to give it some time to be quiet." These words assumed new meaning as I myself experienced "the change."

I especially want to acknowledge Judith Hanson Lasater, Ph.D., P.T., who introduced me to the value of restorative yoga through her workshops and her book, *Relax and Renew: Restful Yoga for Stressful Times.*

I offer one hundred sun salutations to Robin Strasser for enlightening me with the videos she produced—*Menopause S.O.S.: Sharing Options and Support.*

Many thanks to my editors at HCI: Nancy Burke, Christine Belleris and Allison Janse. Also thanks to Kathy Grant, Kim Weiss, Randee Feldman and the sales staff. I could not have finished this book without my photographer, Ruth Miller, and my editorial team on the home front, Anne Gilman; David Moody, Ph.D.; Carin Seebold; Debbie Watson, R.N., B.S.N.; and Christine Golden. Thanks also to my MBA typist and friend Susan Clark (a.k.a. Kali JR). To a writer with one hopeless finger, there is no sweeter music than the heavenly sound of her fingers flying over the keyboard at lightning speed. I thank Paulette Mahurin, R.N., my YOGOpher/errand girl; my son and daughter, Bo and Monica Hebenstreit; and my parents, Rene and Mary Diets. Without their help, I might have fallen off the menopausal bridge. And special love and thanks to Malchia Olshan and Dale Hanson, who are truly the Wise Woman sages in my life.

Introduction

Welcome to Yoga and the Wisdom of Menopause

This is a book about the relationship between the practice of yoga and the wisdom of menopause. It explores how yoga works to support the health and spiritual awakening of women during this important midlife transition and the years that follow.

Today more women than at any time in history are either approaching or in the midst of menopause. Within the next twenty years, between 40 to 60 million women in the United States and an estimated 575 million women worldwide will enter their menopausal years.

As we redefine ourselves as women and face new challenges and responsibilities, our need for solitude, reflection and a spiritual practice increases. Yoga's approach to holistic health is a powerful tool for helping us experience the passage into menopause as a positive event, both physically and spiritually. For those of us wanting to break free of lifelong negative habits and addictions and live life as consciously as possible, practicing yoga provides strength and support. Yoga reduces the effects of menopause's hormonal changes by balancing the endocrine system. It smoothes out the hormonal and glandular changes that take place during this period. Not only does regular practice of yoga ease the physical aspects of menopause, it also inspires a spiritual awakening that helps women open to the power and beauty of this profound change.

Menopause is a natural life event. Long misunderstood in our culture, menopause is as important in the feminine life cycle as menstruation and

At this juncture, practice of yoga asanas is extremely beneficial, as it calms the nervous system and brings equipoise.

—Geeta S. Iyengar,
Yoga: A Gem for Women

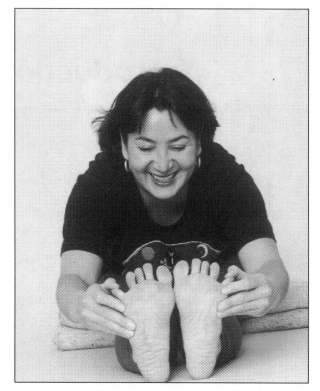

Suza Francina. "Yoga can help us move joyfully into the second half of our lives."

pregnancy. Just as the onset of the menstrual cycle signals the passage from girl to woman, menopause marks a woman's passage to Wise Woman elder.

At around age forty, a woman's body begins to prepare for the menopausal transition. As many wise women have discovered, this is much more than a physical transition from the childbearing to the non-childbearing years.

Ancient matriarchal cultures and many of today's indigenous cultures have long recognized the wisdom of menopause. In Native American traditions, it was only upon entering menopause that women were ready to become the medicine women and shamans of their tribes. Menopause was the initiation into the Wise-Woman stage of life.

Menopause is an opportunity for the fullest blossoming of a woman's power, wisdom and creativity. It is a bridge to a new phase of life when many women report feeling more confident, empowered and energized. Menopause is a metamorphosis, a complete change at the cellular level.

The spiritual science of yoga recognizes that equilibrium in the physical body helps bring emotional balance and mental clarity. Yoga supports a new archetype that depicts older women as wise, strong, healthy and intuitive. When a woman experiences a sense of harmony with her physical being as well as her deeper emotional and spiritual self, she is better prepared to enter the final initiation of her sacred woman's power—menopause.

Contrary to the old medical paradigm that viewed menopause as a hormone deficiency disease, the menopause transition is actually a vital developmental stage. It ushers in the springtime of the second half of life and is often accompanied by surges in creativity and vitality.

Dr. Christiane Northrup, M.D., considers this stage of life "the biggest opportunity for growth and empowerment since adolescence." In her book, *The Wisdom of Menopause,* she writes, "At midlife, more psychic energy becomes available to us than at any time since adolescence. If we strive to work in active partnership with that organic energy, trusting it to help us uncover the unconscious and self-destructive beliefs about ourselves that have held us back from what we could become, then we will find that we have access to

> If we realize that the body event of menopause is connected to a soul event, then it gives more meaning to this transition.
> —Felicity Green, yoga teacher

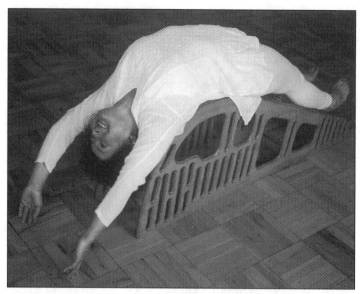

Supported backbend poses tone all the systems of the body during menopause and give a sense of inner joy and happiness.

everything we need to reinvent ourselves as healthier, more resilient women, ready to move joyfully into the second half of our lives."

The word *yoga* comes from the Sanskrit verb *yug,* meaning "to yoke" or "to unite." Yoga is a "unification" of physiological, psychological and spiritual therapies. It is a healing science that addresses all the concerns of women going through menopause.

Yoga teaches that the years after midlife are an ideal time for psychological and spiritual growth. Practicing yoga not only helps us restore health and vitality to our bodies during menopause and the years that follow, but it also supports our emotional and spiritual well-being as we grow older.

During menopause and beyond, there is a shift in what is meaningful and important in our lives. There is a natural movement away from the dictates and expectations of family and society, and an increasing pull inward toward listening to what is important at the level of the soul. Yoga supports and encourages this natural movement to look within rather than seeking answers and validation from the outside.

During menopause, there is also a tremendous shift and release of energy, which can be both unsettling and liberating. The practice of yoga helps us to integrate and cooperate fully with this process. Yoga supports our physical and spiritual journey through menopause.

Yoga practitioners validate what research in women's health has also discovered: Menopause can be profoundly empowering if seen as a spiritual opportunity.

Yoga teacher Judith Lasater (whose story follows this Introduction) reminds us that, "The most valuable thing we can learn from a yoga practice is to change our perspective." A regular yoga practice can help with our attitude toward the whole process of menopause. A well-rounded yoga practice includes an understanding of yoga philosophy, meditation and *pranayama* (regulating the breath) in addition to yoga postures. It encourages a woman to develop an empowered, detached state of mind where she can learn to evaluate herself and her life circumstances without judgment.

Why I Am Writing This Book

Since the publication in 1997 of *The New Yoga for People Over 50,* readers have sent me more comments and questions on yoga and menopause than on any other topic. The chapter on menopause has been widely excerpted, quoted on dozens of Web sites and used as a reprint by teachers for their yoga and menopause workshops.

As women found me on the Web, I began receiving letters from all over the world, letters filled with experiences and questions on yoga and menopause. I was amazed one morning to open my e-mail and find a letter from Tanzania. The writer said:

Dear Ms. Francina,

I am forty-eight years old and started my menopause a year ago. I live in Dar es Salaam, which is in Tanzania, in East Africa. Being near the sea our climate is hot and humid throughout the year. I have been living here for the past two years, and I am suffering even now with hot flushes. The health care system is not the best, and I really don't want to get on HRT [hormone replacement therapy]. I want to go through my menopause as naturally as possible. Please—can you suggest some yoga positions (in detail) which I can follow. I am a healthy person, my weight is normal and I am a vegetarian.

I look forward to hearing from you,
Kind regards,
Najma Chaudry

What really made this letter amazing was the fact that by some strange coincidence my roommate was scheduled to fly to Najma's hometown that very same week! She was able to hand deliver my yoga book with the instructions Najma requested. Talk about synchronicity!

Letters such as this reminded me of how we are all connected in some strange and mysterious way, and that menopause is a universal experience among women the world over.

Another among my e-mails was one from Paddy

O'Brien, a yoga teacher in England and author of several books on yoga for women. She wrote:

> *In terms of my own yoga practice during meno-*
> *pause, for two or three years I've been* confused, *and*
> *your book* really helped *reground and revive me.*
> *Thank you! I have tried the lovely and exciting*
> *Astanga yoga, and Bikram Choudhury's asana*
> *sequence, and they are both marvelous. But I found*
> *myself trudging up the stairs to the small strip of car-*
> *pet by my bed where I practice, feeling like I was*
> *going to cry, and thinking,* I can't do it. I'm too tired.
>
> *I started to feel very old. And to feel (and get!) very*
> *fat. Horrid little injuries plagued me. I got preoccu-*
> *pied with how I "ought" to be able to do this or that*
> *spectacular pose after all these years, and believed*
> *that my inability to do so proved that I was a failure.*
>
> *Finally, thank goodness, I gave up, and just lay*
> *down with my legs up the wall, as you recommend,*
> *and accepted the tiredness for what it is—which is*
> *fairly simple. I have brought up five children while*
> *simultaneously working outside the home. The oldest*
> *is twenty-nine; the youngest is nine and doing most*
> *things for herself now, and finally, I have the space to*
> *feel the tiredness.*
>
> *Since then, my practice has begun to grow again*
> *from the ground up—still shaky, but with hope in it!!*
> *And maybe it will lead to teaching again. I am in one*
> *of those weird transitional times that menopausal*
> *women have where you are on a flat, barren plain with*
> *no map, and even the most frantic efforts (and believe*
> *me, I've made them) will not produce a map or a plan.*
> *I am learning to sit it out, let time pass and wait. For a*
> *let's-get-on-with-it do-er, that's a real learning process.*

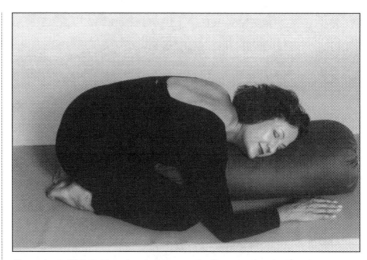

Supported Child's Pose is soothing and relieves stress during the change.

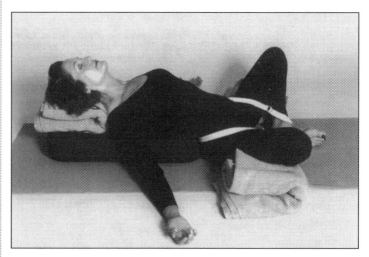

Supported Lying Down Bound Angle Pose (The Goddess Pose) is a key healing and deeply nourishing pose during the menopause transition.

When I read Paddy O'Brien's letter I began to realize that one of the most valuable things a book on yoga and menopause could do is let each of us know that we are not alone in how we feel. This is indeed a time that your body needs extra rest and tender loving care, and you should adjust your yoga practice to help your body through the change rather than fighting it.

When I started skipping periods—which up until then had been as regular as the cycles of the moon—I felt a deep sadness welling up from my very core. I knew this signaled that one phase of my life was coming to an end.

I immersed myself in all the books and tapes on menopause I had collected over the years. Words that had previously been about a far-off event now took on new meaning.

Yoga and the Wisdom of Menopause reflects my own personal experience with menopause, as well as my thirty years of practicing and teaching yoga to women. Many of my women students began practicing yoga at midlife or later. My purpose in writing this book is to illuminate the process we call menopause and shed as much light as possible on this subject from a yogic and spiritual point of view.

How This Book Can Help You

My classes have always been filled with women who began yoga at a time when they were experiencing the physical symptoms of menopause. These symptoms included fatigue, insomnia, headaches, depression, moodiness and hot flashes. Symptoms also often included menstrual problems such as irregular and excessive bleeding. In addition, many of my students came to class with questions about their bone density tests, as well as other serious health concerns such as heart disease and cancer. *Yoga and the Wisdom of Menopause* addresses all these topics.

In this book you will learn how practicing yoga can help you:

- Balance hormonal changes
- Relieve hot flashes, night sweats and other symptoms
- Support pelvic health and cope with common problems such as heavy and irregular bleeding and fibroids
- Alleviate stress and its related physical and emotional symptoms
- Relieve anxiety, mood swings, depression and fatigue
- Strengthen bones and reduce bone loss
- Create cardiovascular health and prevent heart disease
- Strengthen your immune system and cope with breast cancer
- Improve your sense of well-being—physically, emotionally, and spiritually

Throughout this book you will also find inspiring photographs, quotes and personal stories from highly regarded teachers and leaders in the field of women's health and spirituality. All of the women in this book are in their menopausal or postmenopausal years.

You will read stories by women who began yoga to ease menopausal symptoms and interviews with teachers on their experience with menopause. Their collective wisdom will inspire you to implement healthy lifestyle changes and to begin including a yoga practice in your life, if you are not already doing so.

You will learn how yoga postures may relieve hot flashes, night sweats and other common symptoms. Yoga's classic Shoulderstand and various safe variations have long been valued for their cooling and calming effects. My students tell me these postures are an effective antidote to hot flashes and other common symptoms. Supported inverted poses and supported backbends are especially nourishing and rejuvenating during this time. All upside-down poses, according to your ability to practice safely, are recommended before, during and after the menopausal years.

The changes we experience in menopause affect not only the reproductive system but also all the systems of the body. Hormonal fluctuations influence the functioning of all vital organs and tissues—our bones, skin, heart, blood and brain. Thus, we will explore yoga's role in relieving anxiety, mood swings, fatigue and depression; preventing and reversing heart disease; enhancing breast health; and preventing breast cancer and many other health concerns associated with menopause.

The "Yoga and the Wisdom of Menopause Practice Guide" in this book (chapter 8) addresses the special needs of women during perimenopause, menopause and postmenopause. The sequences of poses in the Practice Guide stimulate the ovaries and pituitary gland to produce more hormones. These postures have a calming, soothing, and quieting effect on the nervous system and, if practiced regularly, help ease menopausal symptoms. They also provide a good foundation on which to build a yoga practice that will help you maintain your well-being during your menopausal years and beyond.

Creating a personal yoga practice during the menopausal years helps assure that we have some regular time to be alone and be quiet. As a spiritual practice, yoga provides a welcome "pause" from the multitude of worldly responsibilities we may find ourselves entangled in at midlife. One of the most common long-ings during the menopausal transition is for solitude. According to Dr. Christiane Northrup and other authori-ties on women's health, we are programmed biologi-cally at this stage of life to withdraw from the outside world for a period of time. This is a time to be free of the distractions that come from mothering and focusing our efforts on others. Menopause is a time when we are meant to take care of ourselves.

I have sometimes joked at the implication of the word "men-o-pause." The wise women we will meet in this book invite us to consider the deeper implication of this word association. Their experiences point out that "the pause" goes beyond a break from sex. They invite us to consider the possibility that we are being urged, both biologically and on a soul level, to pause from every-one—to pause from our daily responsibilities—and take some much needed quiet time just to be with ourselves.

I have found that not honoring this deep spiritual need is a great source of stress in the lives of many women. It is no secret that women are the caregivers of the world and have spent their lives juggling outside jobs with homemaking, while caring for children, other family members and an assortment of pets. Most have had little time for solitude, deep rest and a disciplined spiritual practice like yoga.

Menopause is indeed a wake-up call to take care of ourselves. Or, as a doctor friend of mine used to say, "Either take time to be healthy or take time to be sick."

Now that I am at midlife and need to pay more atten-tion to replenishing my own energy reserves, my appre-ciation for yoga's rejuvenating, restorative postures has deepened immeasurably. At this menopausal transition,

I am more grateful then ever for the great gift of yoga. Yoga's healing postures provide me with much needed physical, psychological and spiritual support. When I feel overwhelmed, tired or depressed, I can count on my yoga practice to lift my spirits and give me a sense of peace. My practice gives me the inner strength and resiliency I need to face my own life with honesty and courage and to handle the complexities and uncertainties of living in today's world. Yoga has helped me embrace my menopause, heal, grow, let go and move on. I want the same for you.

The years ahead will no doubt bring dramatic changes in how our society views menopause and older women. Alternative or complementary therapies, Eastern philosophy, as well as new understandings of the biology, psychology and spirituality of the feminine life cycle are moving into the mainstream.

It is my hope that this book will serve as a guide to yoga during menopause for new and experienced practitioners and will also serve to encourage those of you who have been thinking about starting a yoga practice to seek out a caring and knowledgeable teacher. Your teacher will help you make yoga a supportive companion during menopause and for the rest of your life.

Namasté,*
Suza Francina
Ojai, California

---

* *Namasté is an Indian gesture of respect, practiced by placing the palms together in prayer position, at the heart center. It is usually accompanied by lightly bowing the head and body. Namasté is a traditional expression of greeting and farewell practiced among yogis. In simplest terms it means, "The divine in me recognizes and honors the divine in you."*

Twentieth-century anthropologist Margaret Mead wrote about "postmenopausal zest," that resurgence of energy which follows the shift in hormonal and reproductive states. It is hopeful to know there is a light at the end of the tunnel. But I assert there is also light in the tunnel—in the fruitful darkness of menopause.

—Judith Lasater, Ph.D., P.T.
Relax & Renew: Restful Yoga for Stressful Times

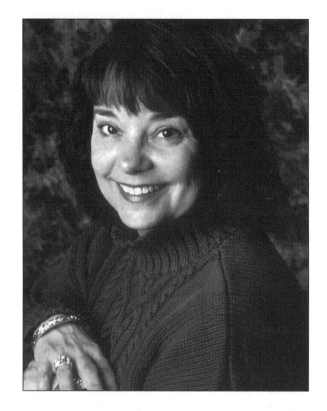

Judith Hanson Lasater, age 55

Menopause Was What Happened to Older Women—Not Me!

I'll never forget my first gray hair. I was in my late thirties, and I felt the stirrings of a rising panic as I stared into the mirror one morning in disbelief. My response was to do what many of us do in these cases: I quickly plucked it out and then happily went into denial. It actually worked well for a while.

But that dose of reality was nothing compared to my introduction a few years later to the process called "perimenopause"—that time before one's periods actually stop completely, but during which lots of interesting symptoms may appear. Pleasantly asleep early one January morning, I suddenly woke up, throwing off the covers as I felt my face flood with heat. Was I sleeping in the hot sun? Who had opened the shades? What was happening to me? The heat soon subsided, and as I lay back, I reflected on what had just occurred. A little voice in my head said, *Now I know what a hot flash feels like,* but my conscious, thinking brain said, *No way. I am too young for that.*

The following morning nothing happened, and I felt smugly free. It must have been an anomaly, I told myself. But over the next few weeks and months, I was to learn that indeed it was not an anomaly. From then on, a couple of mornings a week, I would be awakened by a little dose of "my own private summer."

I definitely felt surprised, but I discounted this experience as everything else in my body felt normal. I did ask an older friend about the symptoms at the beginning of menopause, and the first thing she mentioned was "mood swings."

"How do I tell?" I asked, and we both laughed.

Eventually I began to admit to myself what was happening, and I started studying about menopause. I began to read everything I could get my hands on and learned that the period of perimenopause that I was beginning could actually last for five years or more.

Startled, I experienced a rush of emotions. No

The ocean is ever-changing, ever-renewing. The waves advance and recede in a predictable rhythm. The water that rushed to shore an hour ago may be many miles out to sea in the present moment. This rhythm is a powerful image for the woman in premenopause. As the roles of young woman and babymaker recede, something new fills the space.
—Judith Lasater, Ph.D., P.T.
Relax & Renew: Restful Yoga for Stressful Times

one had ever told me about perimenopause. I had always believed that practicing yoga *asanas, pranayama* (breathing exercises) and meditation would somehow "protect" me against many health issues. One day I would just stop having my periods and that would be that. But I was learning that even a long-standing and focused yoga practice could not protect me against the inevitability of life changes and the passage of time.

I went through a period of disbelief. Menopause was what happened to "older" women, not me. Yes, I was still in my forties, albeit my late forties, but I was full of energy. Besides, I could stand on my hands in the center of the room! How could this be happening to me?

Over the next couple of years, other changes began to manifest in my body and psyche. But now, unlike that first hot flash, my reading had prepared me for them. I was deeply thankful also for the knowledge, wisdom and counsel of other women, as well as for the gift of my own yoga practice to ground me. Besides the occasional hot flash, luckily I was sailing right through this time of my life with very few symptoms.

By trial and error I learned which poses helped me feel more like myself, and I settled on a practice heavily centered around supported backbends, supported inversions and many restorative poses. These poses seemed to even out my energy and reduce moodiness.

The next five years were full of work I loved,

books to be written, workshops to be taught, more traveling with my husband, and involvement with my three teenagers as they became young adults and made those exciting life decisions like college choice. Through it all, I came back again and again to my yoga mat, specifically for solace and balancing. I also found that I was beginning to "crave" a meditation practice, and for the first time this became a regular and "never miss" daily practice.

Along with this, things seemed to even out in my body. I discovered natural progesterone and estrogen creams, and I found an application schedule and dose that worked for me. I discovered that if I missed my application for a few days, the hot flashes would occur.

Now even those have gone, and in their place is the barest beginning of a spontaneous calmness. I am less ruffled by it all. And I feel a depth of compassion for myself and others that I did not experience in my youth. Then I was pushing myself to teach lots of classes and workshops, and raise three young children—all while getting up early for my own yoga practice and then staying up late to write articles for *Yoga Journal* magazine.

I feel lucky that I had the gift of yoga *asana* and yoga philosophy in my life long before the physical and emotional changes of perimenopause and menopause were upon me. I have had choices. I trust my body, and I am dedicated to being present with my life as it unfolds. Given that context, I am enjoying this new stage of my life. In fact, I am

> The practice of yoga is fundamentally an act of kindness toward oneself.
> —Judith Lasater, Ph.D., P.T.
> *Living Your Yoga: Finding the Spiritual in Everyday Life*

beginning to think of it as just another "asana."

Judith Hanson Lasater, Ph.D., and physical therapist, a respected and internationally known yoga teacher, has taught yoga since 1971. She writes extensively on the therapeutic aspects of yoga and is the author of Relax and Renew: Restful Yoga for Stressful Times *and* Living Your Yoga: Finding the Spiritual in Everyday Life, *both from Rodmell Press, Berkeley, California.*

1 The Yoga of Menopause: Alternatives to Hormone Therapy

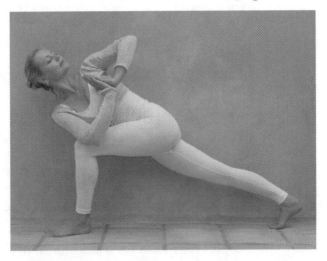

At midlife, the hormonal milieu that was present for only a few days each month during most of your reproductive years, the milieu that was designed to spur you on to re-examine your life just a little at a time, now gets stuck in the on position for weeks or months at a time. We go from an alternating current of inner wisdom to a direct current that remains on all the time after menopause is complete. During perimenopause, our brains make the change from one way of being to the other.

—CHRISTIANE NORTHRUP, M.D., *THE WISDOM OF MENOPAUSE: CREATING PHYSICAL AND EMOTIONAL HEALTH AND HEALING DURING THE CHANGE*

Woman's lives are deeply affected by the ebb and flow of their hormones—those mysterious and miraculous molecules that deliver vital messages via the bloodstream from one part of the body to another. Indeed, our lives are patterned by the cycles of nature, whether these are the changes of puberty, the monthly rhythms of our menstrual cycle or the passages of menopause. These changes have undisputed effects on our whole being. No woman can menstruate, give birth or cross the menopausal bridge without feeling these hormonal influences on her physical, emotional and psychological state.

Yoga's Unique Benefits During the Menopausal Years

Achieving hormonal balance during the menopausal years is essential to good health. Among the many benefits that set yoga apart from other forms of physical exercise is the effect yoga postures and breathing practices have not only on the muscles and bones of your body, but also on your organs and glands. In this book we explain the effect that these postures can have on your hormonal system, and how to use yoga to work with your body as it goes through hormonal and other changes during menopause.

Practicing yoga can help prevent or reduce the common symptoms that affect women specifically during the menopausal years by providing a form of treatment directed at the root causes that result in the breakdown of the healthy functioning of the body.

It's important to bear in mind that all menopausal symptoms are related, and using yoga to ease the unpleasant effect of one symptom generally leads to better health in the rest of the body. Every yoga pose has a multitude of effects on all the systems of the body.

The experiences of longtime yoga practitioners show that certain poses and sequences of poses act as a tonic for the healthy functioning of certain body systems or organs. Equally important for your health during menopause is the overall positive effect of yoga on the body as a whole.

The regular practice of all the categories of poses—standing, sitting, lying down, backbends, forward bends, twists and inverted (upside down) poses—stimulates and activates all the glands, organs, tissues and cells of the body. Yoga's inverted poses are particularly important during menopause, as they have a powerful effect on the neuroendocrine system, allowing fresh, oxygenated blood to flow to the glands in the head and neck. In each yoga posture (asana), different organs and glands are placed in various anatomical positions and are supplied with fresh blood, gently massaged, relaxed, toned and stimulated.

Yoga's approach to health during menopause and beyond is based on the premise that the body should be allowed to function as efficiently, effectively and naturally as possible. Practicing the postures recommended for the menopause transition, in a way that is appropriate for your present physical and emotional condition, will gradually rejuvenate your body and remove the causes of unpleasant symptoms that you may be experiencing.

What Is Menopause?

A woman's life unfolds in three major physical stages that are determined by her reproductive system. In her

When we complete menopause we move beyond the alternating cyclic nature and become like a direct current, charged and focused with the ability to speak and act truth and to express directly who we are through our inner vision. Certainly there is a tremendous shift of energy that is both liberating and powerful. We need to cooperate fully with this process to make the most of this creative opportunity.
—Farida Sharan, N.D., *Creative Menopause: Illuminating Women's Health and Spirituality*

The time has come for us to reclaim menopause from those who try to define it for us—and to look squarely at those who wish to medicalize it.

—Susan M. Love, M.D., Dr. Susan Love's Hormone Book: Making Informed Choices About Menopause

childhood, before the onset of menses, she is in the "maiden" stage. After puberty, in her childbearing years, she is biologically in the "mother" phase of life, even if she chooses not to have children. At approximately midlife, production of estrogen and progesterone by the ovaries slows down. Menstruation becomes irregular and eventually ends. The years immediately preceding and following the last menstrual period are called the menopausal years, or climacteric or crest. A year or so after menstruation stops is the beginning of the third major stage of a woman's life—the "crone" or "Wise Woman" stage.

The word "menopause" is from the Greek words *men* or *meno* for "month" and *pausis* for "pause" or "stop." Simply stated, menopause is the cessation of menstrual periods, an end to the monthly cycle.

Menopause has three stages. The first stage is perimenopause, which literally means "premenopause," a change in hormonal functions leading up to menopause. Perimenopause occurs typically around age forty, but it can begin in the thirties when the menstrual cycle is still normal. It can last as long as fifteen years, but on average lasts around five years. This is the time during which women notice changes in their periods from lighter and longer to heavier and more frequent. The greatest fluctuations in hormones occur during perimenopause, and this stage is often described as puberty in reverse.

The second stage, menopause itself, is actually the cessation of menstruation (menses). Menopause is considered official twelve months after the last period. The average age of women whose menstrual periods have stopped is fifty-two. Although a woman may no longer be having any periods, her emotions can still fluctuate. Hot flashes, or "power surges" as many women prefer to call them, may still be present, and the body is still adjusting to the change in hormone levels. This period can last several more years.

The final stage, which lasts the remainder of a woman's life, is postmenopause. At this point, a woman's body is generally comfortable and has adjusted to its hormone levels.

Hormones 101

Women crossing the menopausal bridge today are living in the midst of an unprecedented, mass scale hormone experiment. Observers of the menopause industry predict we will look back on this era, when millions of women swallowed a drug derived from the urine of pregnant mares, as one of the biggest medical fiascos ever. While I was in the midst of writing this book, news was released that a branch of the Woman's Health Initiative Study had been stopped earlier than anticipated. Their research established that women taking PremPro, a combination of Premarin and Provera, were found to have increased risk of invasive breast cancer, heart attack, stroke and blood clots in the lungs.

Many experts still claim the risk is minimal. Women considering hormone replacement therapy (HRT) need to educate themselves about the different types of hormones available. There are many excellent books listed in the Resource section that provide in-depth discussions of hormones. Among the ones I recommend for their holistic approaches to women's health are: *The Wisdom of Menopause,* by Christiane Northrup, M.D.;

We stand at the confluence of profound changes. Our present medical system is symptom-fixated and driven by misplaced economic incentives, but now faces stiff competition from alternative practitioners. Women's health problems clustered under the banner of hormone balance are epidemic and not well addressed by mainstream medicine. Women are emerging from under a cloud of historic medical neglect and are rightly demanding new and more effective approaches.
—John R. Lee, M.D., *What Your Doctor May Not Tell You About Menopause—The Breakthrough Book on Natural Progesterone*

Menopause is a metamorphosis, like a caterpillar becoming a butterfly. The caterpillar needs a cocoon, and so do you. One of the most important things you can do during menopause is to take time for you. Go into your cave, go into your cocoon, go into your room and shut the door.

—Susun S. Weed,
The Menopausal Years: The Wise Woman Way

Dr. Susan Love's Hormone Book, by Susan M. Love, M.D.; *What Your Doctor May Not Tell You About Menopause,* by John R. Lee, M.D.; *Hormone Heresy,* by Sherrill Sellman; and *Menopause: Bridging the Gap Between Natural and Conventional Medicine,* by Lorilee Schoenbeck, N.D.

Yoga poses that turn the body halfway or completely upside down, such as Standing Forward Bends, Downward-Facing Dog and various inverted poses, stimulate the endocrine system, especially the pituitary gland. This small gland in the center of the brain is involved in the regulation of blood-sugar levels and body temperature, and controls the changes in the hormone levels that occur in menopause.

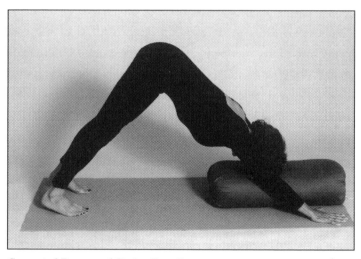

Supported Downward-Facing Dog Pose.

Menopause as Metamorphosis

Susun Weed, in her book, *The Menopausal Years: The Wise Woman Way,* describes menopause as a metamorphosis, a complete change at the cellular level, where a woman changes from one person to another, similar to the dramatic change that occurs during puberty. Susun Weed and other holistic healers who have studied the ancient women's mysteries remind us of the power and initiation potential of these two unique life events: menstruation and menopause. She views the menopausal years as the years of transformation from a potential mother to Wise Woman elder or crone.

Forward bends also gently compress the abdomen, massaging the uterus and other abdominal organs. When we come out of the pose and release the compression, the organs are bathed in freshly oxygenated blood, and we feel refreshed and rejuvenated. This alternate squeezing and soaking enhances the functioning of the ovaries and the hormones they produce. Forward bends also soothe the nervous system and have a quieting effect on the mind.

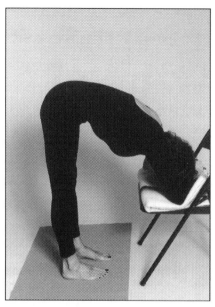

Standing Forward Bend Pose with head resting on chair helps to relax the brain and nervous system.

A Word on Weight Gain During Menopause

Women almost universally experience weight gain during the menopausal years. Maybe that is nature's wisdom. The two ways the body produces its own natural hormones after the menstrual cycle stops are from body fat and the adrenal glands.

We need a certain amount of fat to produce our own hormones. We store excess estrogen in our fat cells. As our estrogen drops, we can call on that extra estrogen to make the menopausal transition easier. Women who are thin, especially if they follow extreme diets to lose weight, tend to have a more difficult menopause.

Some researchers believe that menopausal weight gain, so long as it is not excessive, is also nature's

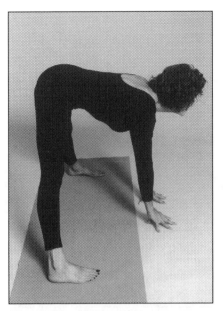

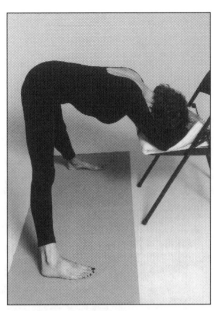

Standing Forward Bends stimulate the endocrine system, especially the pituitary gland, which controls the changes in hormones that occur in menopause.

Wide Angle Standing Forward Bend Pose with head supported.

protection against thinning bones. Researchers have found that adequate body fat improves bone density. Women who are a little heavier than the dictates of this culture's impossibly thin standards may actually experience an easier transition during the menopausal years due in part to excess estrogen stores in fat cells.

Since yoga stimulates the muscles, bones and endocrine system, it tends to balance your metabolism and allows the natural intelligence of your body to determine your physical shape.

Key Poses to Help Balance Your Hormones

See chapter 8, "Yoga and the Wisdom of Menopause Practice Guide," for instructions.

Note on time: Do not be in a hurry. Select only the number of poses you can do without feeling rushed. **Time suggested is the minimum time.** Experienced practitioners can stay in poses longer.

Pose	Suggested Time
Wide Angle Standing Forward Bend with Head Supported	1 minute
Standing Forward Bend with Head Supported	1 minute
Supported Downward-Facing Dog Pose	1 minute
Hanging Downward-Facing Dog Pose	1 minute
Supported Lying Down Bound Angle Pose	10 minutes
Supported Legs Up the Wall Pose	10 minutes
Supported Bridge Pose	5 to 10 minutes
Deep Relaxation Pose with Bolster Under Legs, Sandbag Across Abdomen	5 to 10 minutes

See also, Key Poses to Ease Hot Flashes, page 91.

Carin Seebold, age 57

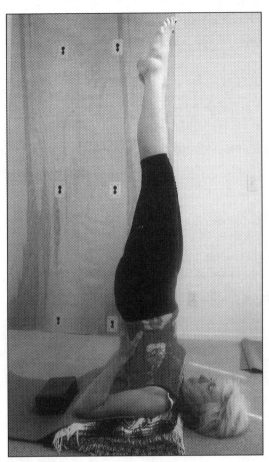

Shoulderstand (Sarvangasana), the queen or mother of all yoga poses.

I Did *Not* Want to Take Hormone Replacement Therapy

Menopause equals depression, dysfunction and debilitation. These were my thoughts some fifteen or twenty years before I reached menopause. A male friend at the time firmly believed all these things and more. He reminded me many times that his family seriously considered institutionalizing his mother when she went through the change. So you can imagine how I dreaded this time of life, secretly fearing for my own sanity.

Looking back, I see how easily misled we can be!

I started perimenopause around fifty-two years of age. Other than erratic periods and depression (aggravated by my mother's passing around the same time), I had few of the symptoms normally associated with the change. Sometimes tiny beads of sweat would gather on my brow with a fleeting feeling of a heated flush—then I was back to normal. I had no night sweats at all.

I was adamant about hormone replacement therapy—I did not want to take it. I had witnessed the difficulty some friends had adjusting to this regimen. My physician never asked me what I wanted. She just wanted to write out a prescription. After all, wasn't I like umpteen hundred women she saw every day going through this period of life? Wasn't it standard procedure to prescribe hormone therapy? Well, it may be for some, but it wasn't for me. I dismissed her recommendation.

Having tired of weight lifting, personal trainers, gyms and water aerobics, I decided at this time—I was fifty-three—to take a yoga class sponsored by parks and recreation. This class met once a week for six weeks, and I liked it so well I repeated it. I was hooked! I moved on to a yoga studio, beginning with once a week and eventually working up to three or four classes a week.

I was avidly reading all the yoga books I could find; I was hungry to learn more about this new passion of mine. I explored the philosophies that accompany yoga practice, including nonviolence, meditation, breathing and healthy eating. A turning point occurred for me when I stumbled upon Suza Francina's book *The New Yoga for People Over 50*. I started attending her classes in Ojai, California, in addition to my regular evening classes.

Practicing yoga made my menopausal transition so easy. I cannot say specifically why or how, but I know this is what made the difference between myself and friends who experienced great difficulty through this important passage. Among other things—before I started yoga—my buttocks seemed to have slipped south, with no end in sight, and my thighs were flopping about no matter how much I exercised them. Regular yoga practice moved my buttocks back where they belonged, and my thighs are again firm with elongated muscles. In addition, my flexibility has increased immeasurably. And if anyone had told me I would be doing headstands and handstands at my age, I would have scoffed at them. But I do, and it feels wonderful!

I am intensely offended at the magazine advertising relative to menopause. If we were to believe what we see in the media, we'd all be dried up, sexually over-the-hill, and "flashing" until we wept. Our bones would be getting weaker by the day as we tried to deal with this "disease" called menopause. Has anyone ever called menstruation a disease? Menopause is a normal transition to the wise old crone stage of life, when we can revel in our independence, seek new directions and work with a body that is flexible and strong.

In addition to the physical benefits, yoga is a wonderful stress reliever and a means of introduction to your inner self. It can lead you down a new and exciting path, one filled with life-affirming possibilities. Yoga and the wisdom of menopause—perfect companions!

Carin Seebold, 57, began yoga at age 53. She continues to expand her knowledge and practice of yoga, holistic medicine and her own spirituality. She enjoys taking yoga vacations, has her own "yoga room" at home and is grateful to her teachers, especially Linda DiCarlo and Suza Francina, for helping her along the path.

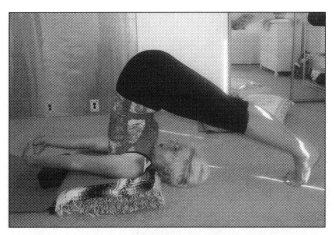

Plow Pose (Halasana) helps balance your endocrine system and quiets your nervous system during menopause.

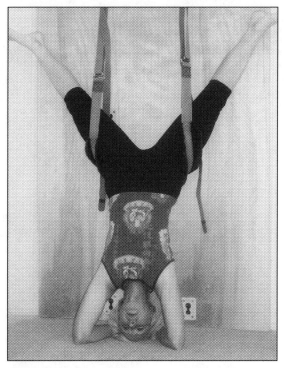

Supported Headstand hanging from a pelvic sling (or ropes) improves the functioning of the endocrine glands. The feeling of increased energy and revitalization in the body and brain that occurs after practicing inversions cannot be overemphasized during menopause.

Sirsasana stimulates the blood supply to the brain and activates the pituitary and pineal glands. The practice of Headstand revitalizes the entire body.

—Geeta S. Iyengar
Yoga: A Gem for Women

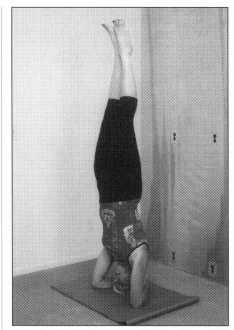

Headstand (**Sirsasana**).

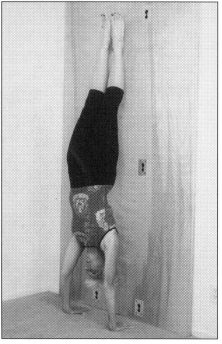

Handstands keep your bones strong and are empowering during menopause.

Gretchen Newmark, age 53

I Found I Needed Hormones!

I never thought about menopause until my very late forties. I was already doing all the things that were suggested to have a "natural menopause," so I assumed that I would have no symptoms and it would be a nonevent. I am a nutritionist, and my diet was what was recommended—low in fat, salt and sugar; high in fiber, vitamins, minerals and phytochemicals. I was taking a high-quality supplement and eating plenty of soy and a few table-spoons of ground flaxseeds everyday. I maintained a regular yoga practice. I was walking for an hour or more five or six times a week. I meditated morning and evening. My stress level was low—I was happily married, loved my work and friends, and I didn't tend to overdo. It looked like a lifestyle that would make menopause a breeze.

When I first began having symptoms, I didn't attribute them to menopause. I was waking up every night at about 2:00 or 3:00 A.M. and could not go back to sleep. I would be exhausted the next day. I tried melatonin but it didn't help. My sex drive diminished to zero. I began to lose my memory and couldn't remember simple names, words or even the end of the sentence I'd begun. My tissues were getting fragile, but neither my naturopathic doctor nor I recognized that the hemorrhoids I developed had anything to do with menopause. I was surprised that the flax oil wasn't helping with vaginal dryness and irritation.

Gradually, my symptoms became less and less tolerable. I was bloated and uncomfortable two weeks of the month. I decided to work with an acupuncturist and take herbs. Still the symptoms didn't improve.

My mood became unpredictable. I found myself feeling rage for no reason and saying and doing things that hurt other people and myself. This was intolerable. I made an appointment with a naturo-pathic physician who was skillful in prescribing natural hormones. I never thought I would resort to hormones. It was against my principles of using only natural approaches. But I felt desperate.

This physician described the benefits of natural hormones. Besides the symptomatic relief, I would be preventing bone loss (I'm small and fair) and brain deterioration. She said that she would pre-scribe the smallest amounts that would do the job. She saw me through the years of perimenopause when my natural hormone levels were erratic. We had to change my prescription as often as once a month. I am deeply indebted to her for giving me a quality of life similar to what it had been before menopause.

I was embarrassed that I was resorting to replacement hormones. My idea of myself as a per-son free of medication was over. To my surprise, however, I found that many of my friends were gradually making the same decision—even two of my yoga teacher friends. Everyone I talked with had found that the natural approaches they were using weren't enough, and that they needed hormones. We began trading names of physicians who prescribed them. I wasn't the only one.

If I could give one piece of advice to women who are facing menopause it would be this: Don't try to predict in advance what it will be like or what you will need. Take advantage of all the natural approaches we are so lucky to have available. If you do find you need hormones, don't think of it as a failure on your part. We are different people with different needs.

Let's celebrate the transition of menopause and all the years we can enjoy after. May we all neither cling to youth nor allow our bodies and minds to deteriorate before their time. May we age gracefully, full of life, wisdom and excitement.

Gretchen Newmark, age 53, taught yoga in Santa Monica, California, and Portland, Oregon, at the Julie Lawrence Yoga Center. She is a nutritionist in private practice, a spiritual director providing ecumenical spiritual counseling and a meditation teacher. She says that being in her fifties is a whole lot of fun so far.

Ingrid Boulting, age 55

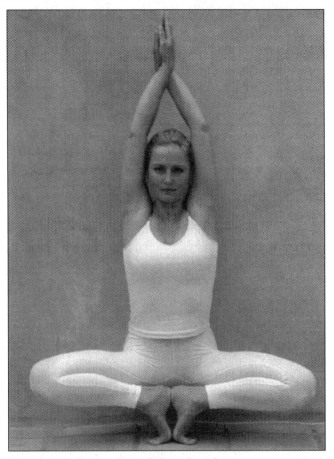

Bound Angle Pose variation balanced on the toes.

Smooth Transition Due to Yoga and Diet

I am fifty-five years old. I still had my period until it came to a sudden end ten months ago. I had regular periods up until then with no problems. I felt fortunate in that I never had cramping or bloating or any of the other symptoms many women seem to suffer from. I have not experienced any hot flashes or other symptoms that can accompany menopause. My sexual life continues to be active and healthy. I believe this smooth transition through menopause was due to my diet and my yoga practice. I have been a vegetarian for thirty-six years. I became a vegetarian for humanitarian reasons first. The many preventive health benefits were another advantage. By cutting out meats and pesticides one avoids ingesting the many hormone disrupters that come along with commercially produced foods.

I started yoga in New York in the early 1970s in search of a deeper understanding of life. Yoga naturally lends itself to living a more natural lifestyle that is in harmony with nature. With a disciplined practice, I found many unwanted habits dropped away effortlessly.

When I was eighteen years old, my English naturopathic doctor, Gordon Latto, told me that vegetarian women have no problems with their periods or with menopause. He said that the toxins and acids from animal products in the blood cause many problems, including cancers. His wife was a living example of a very healthy and vibrant seventy-year-old vegetarian who was a positive role model for me.

I also know that yoga has a powerful effect on balancing all the systems of the body, including the endocrine system. I could feel the many health benefits from my regular practice and this inspired me to become a yoga teacher. I had suffered from an underactive thyroid gland. The doctor wanted to give me hormones. I did yoga instead and included kelp in my diet. The problem corrected itself. My grandmother never took hormones. They did not exist in her time, and she survived menopause. I eat mostly raw organic foods, sprouted seeds and nuts and vegetable juices. I gave up drinking coffee as much as I loved it because it is a known endocrine disrupter. One of my intentions in my yoga practice was to be as healthy as possible so that my spiritual and creative life could thrive. Yoga and a healthy vegetarian diet really work. I can highly recommend it.

Namasté

Ingrid Boulting is a yoga teacher at Sacred Space Studio, in Ojai, California. She started studying yoga in 1972 under the guidance of Sachidananda. She has continued her own practice through the years, studying the various traditions of yoga, and incorporates the best of all of them in her teachings.

2 Yoga and the Endocrine System

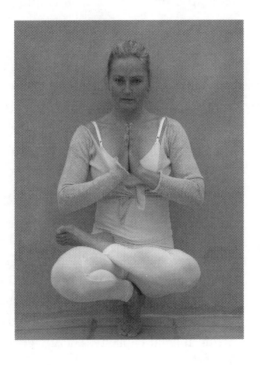

Sometimes, rest is the highest spiritual practice.

—Tom Yeomans, psychologist and poet

*Plan rest into your life as surely as you
plan exercise into it, and make it
as delicious as you can.*

—Paddy O'Brien, *Becoming Yourself*

A woman's physical well-being during the menopausal years depends on the healthy functioning of her endocrine (hormone-producing) glands. In order to understand just how important the endocrine system is during menopause, it is helpful to have some basic information about its structure and function.

Comprised of small bits of tissue, the endocrine (meaning "in pouring") glands are internal secretion— or ductless—glands. They differ from external secretion glands, such as sweat or tear glands, because they secrete substances directly into the bloodstream rather than pouring them out through a tube or duct. The substances secreted by the endocrine glands are called hormones, also described as "biochemical messengers" of the blood.

Hormones, even in extremely tiny amounts, are unbelievably potent; they direct and regulate much of the subtle biochemistry of life. They are distributed to all parts of the body and have tremendous influence not only on our physical bodies, but also on our temperament, mental capacity, energy, personality and outlook on life.

A woman's body is quite capable of adjusting to the hormonal changes that occur when the ovaries slow down. The sex hormones—estrogen, progesterone and the androgens—are produced in body fat, skin, the brain, the adrenal glands and other sites besides the ovaries, as the need arises. If all our other glands are functioning well, they will, in most cases, continue to produce all the hormones a woman needs for the rest of her life.

The Endocrine Glands

The major glands of the endocrine system are: the pituitary gland, imbedded deep in the skull at the base of the brain; the hypothalamus, a region of the brain that lies just above the pituitary; the pineal gland, also located near the pituitary; the butterfly-shaped thyroid gland at the base of the neck (the throat region); the parathyroid glands, located behind the thyroid; the islets of Langerhans, in the pancreas; the two adrenal glands located above the right and left kidneys; and the two almond-shaped ovaries located in the bowl of the pelvis.

The thyroid gland, the comparative giant in size, weighs approximately one ounce; the parathyroids are so tiny that they are scarcely visible; the adrenal glands are about the size of a small lima bean; and the pituitary is about half an inch long—the size of a pea. The pituitary controls the function of most other endocrine glands and is, in turn, controlled by the hypothalamus. As the master gland, the pituitary regulates the other glands and performs important functions of its own, including those governing a woman's reproductive cycle.

The hypothalamus controls and integrates parts of the nervous system and endocrine processes, and many bodily functions such as temperature, sleep and appetite.

The functions of the pineal gland are not yet fully understood by modern science, but some yogis and other mystics believe that there is a strong connection between the pineal gland and our spiritual life.

Science *has* discovered that the pineal gland is affected by exposure to light and seasonal changes, which appear to regulate rhythms of fertility and sexual activity. The pineal gland produces a hormone called melatonin, as well as other substances, which influence the health of the immune system.

The ancient yogis believed that the pineal gland secretes a special fluid or nectar—called *amrita*—which is important to longevity. Turning the body upside down helps increase and retain this regenerative substance. Naturopath Farida Sharan writes in *Creative Menopause* that, "The pineal gland responds to the influence of the cosmos, the stars, the plants, seasons . . . colors, vibrations, sound and light, connecting the macrocosm of universal destiny to the microcosm of our personal destiny."

The islets of Langerhans are clusters of endocrine cells located in the pancreas that secrete insulin. Their principal function is to regulate carbohydrate metabolism—that is, blood sugar level, which is vital to our overall health, mood and energy. When we ingest sugar, our blood sugar level goes up. The islets of Langerhans detect this excess sugar in the blood and secrete insulin, which brings the blood sugar level back to normal.

The ovaries are the female equivalent of the male testes. They are an important producer of androgens, the hormones involved in normal sex drive. Normal menopause, with ovaries and uterus intact, is a natural physiological event that takes place over a period of several years. As the ovaries gradually retire from producing eggs, the adrenal glands and other organs take over some hormone production, as does body fat and other body sites. During menopause, the ovaries secrete smaller and smaller amounts of estrogen and progesterone, and egg release (ovulation) eventually stops.

All the glands in the endocrine system work together. Each gland has an influence on all the others, and the interactions of the various hormones are vital to the health of the whole endocrine system. Because these glands secrete hormones directly into the bloodstream, they have the capacity to respond to emergencies in a matter of seconds, directing the various systems of the body into action.

Although these powerful glands are relatively small compared to the body's organs and muscles, they have far-reaching effects on every physiological function of the body. Any disorder in even one gland can have serious repercussions for the body's health.

Yoga, Menopause and Thyroid Function

According to Christiane Northrup, M.D., and John R. Lee, M.D., thyroid problems are very common during the perimenopausal and postmenopausal years. Estrogen, progesterone and thyroid hormones are interrelated. The thyroid gland regulates your metabolism, stimulates growth and helps protect the body from infection. Among the most common menopausal symptoms connected to thyroid function are mood disturbances (most often seen in the form of depression and irritability), low energy level, constipation, cold intolerance, weight gain, mental confusion and sleep disturbances. Many yoga poses, especially the Shoulderstand, are well known for improving the functioning of the thyroid and parathyroid gland.

The Adrenal Glands: Mood Swings and Fatigue

While the ovaries decrease their production of androgenic hormones (the hormones associated with sexual responsiveness and a general sense of well-being) during

Your health is more important than all the things you have to do. . . . Remember, you are worth it.
—Elise Browning Miller, *Life Is a Stretch*

Menopause is a time
for taking stock, of
spiritual as well as
physical change, and it
would be a pity to be
unconscious of it.
—Germaine Greer,
*The Change: Women,
Aging and Menopause*

menopause, other parts of the body, such as the pineal and adrenal glands, actually increase their hormonal output.

Because the adrenal glands can partially take over for the ovaries and must now produce the small amount of estrogen the body needs to keep functioning properly, healthy adrenal glands are crucial for negotiating the menopausal transition. Unfortunately, for many midlife and older women, the adrenals are depleted by habitual stress, poor nutrition, constant stimulation from substances like sugar and coffee, environmental pollution and other problems. Depleted adrenal glands may produce mood swings, fatigue or depression—all symptoms that are commonly attributed to menopause.

The two thumb-sized adrenal glands are comprised of two components and secrete three essential hormones. The adrenal medulla secretes epinephrine (adrenaline) and norepinephrine (noradrenaline). These hormones make your heart pound, raise your blood pressure, help make your muscles tense and put your brain on high alert. The adrenal cortex secretes cortisol and other hormones. Cortisol is a natural steroid that suppresses inflammation and raises your blood-sugar level so that your muscles have plenty of fuel. Cortisol also *suppresses* the immune system.

The adrenal hormones are catabolic, which means that they foster biological processes that burn energy and break down cellular structures. If you activate the adrenal glands repeatedly without sufficient recovery in between, your body becomes depleted and exhausted. You become susceptible to mood swings, depression and other illnesses connected to chronic fatigue. Coffee, sugar and other stimulants can all exacerbate mood swings at any stage of life, but most especially during menopause.

The Adrenal Hormones and Tolerating Stress

The adrenal hormones help us tolerate many of the stresses and burdens of life. However, many women—possibly even the vast majority—enter menopause with their adrenals already exhausted from years of juggling the responsibilities of family and work outside the home. If life has been chronically stressful or if you have been ill, then you have asked your adrenal glands to work overtime and have not given them adequate time to replenish themselves.

Stress is now recognized as one of the foremost contributors to ill health, and uncomfortable menopausal symptoms are no exception. Your mind and body will function more efficiently during all the stages of life, including menopause, if stress is removed.

According to stress expert Hans Selye, M.D., stress triggers three distinct stages or reactions: the Alarm Reaction Stage of hyperfunctioning adrenals with excess hormones; the Resistance Stage, which stimulates adrenal adaptation, drawing energy and nutrients from reserves (i.e., the body adapts to living in a state of chronic stress); and the Exhaustion Stage, where both the body's energy and nutritional reserves are depleted, causing chronic fatigue.

Common symptoms of adrenal exhaustion include fatigue, low stamina, depression, mood swings and addiction to coffee and sugar. (Note that mood swings are even more exacerbated during menopause by substances that stimulate and then crash the adrenals, like coffee and sugar.) Adrenal exhaustion symptoms are frequently confused as menopausal symptoms because hyper-functioning adrenals can cause hot flashes,

> We cannot over-estimate the role that stress plays in making menstrual and menopausal symptoms worse.
> —Larry Payne, Ph.D., Richard Usatine, M.D., *Yoga Rx*

headaches, dizziness, high blood pressure, facial and body hair growth and other changes associated with estrogen deficiency. Many women have observed that drinking coffee, which results in adrenal stimulation, increases sweat gland activity, which may contribute to night sweats.

Krishna Raman, M.D., who studied yoga with the great yoga master B.K.S. Iyengar, writes in his ground-breaking book, *A Matter of Health: Integration of Yoga and Eastern Medicine for Prevention and Cure,* that decreased adrenal activity—a common endocrine dysfunction—is responsible for lack of energy. He states:

If the adrenal gland is well massaged every day by asanas, such changes will not occur. The health of the individual cells of the gland is toned up by yoga. Stimulation of the glands provides greater energy than before. Standing poses invigorate the glands. Inversions recharge the adrenals. Twisting asanas are invaluable for rinsing the adrenal glands. Backbends squeeze the adrenals. Forward bends soothe the overdrive. Half Halasana relieves the overdrive. Energy levels depend principally on healthy endocrine and nervous functions. Yoga interacts in these areas by stabilizing the inner vital life force in the body.

Constantly stimulating the adrenals, whether through coffee, sugar, salt or excessive exercise and various "charged" activities, is like beating a tired horse. Far wiser is to let the horse out to pasture and give her time to rest and rejuvenate.

Yoga for Adrenal Health

Yoga helps modulate mood swings and reduce depression and anxiety by helping to balance a woman's changing hormones. Many of the symptoms commonly associated with menopause, such as irritability, depression, and various aches and pains, are intensified by the inability to cope with stress. Practicing yoga's relaxing, restorative poses on a regular basis helps ease these symptoms. Equally important, yoga practice gives you the opportunity to weed out and clear away the mental and emotional debris that is the root cause of many problems associated with menopause.

Yoga's relaxing, rejuvenating inverted poses and other important restorative poses can break the vicious cycle of adrenal exhaustion, stimulation and fatigue. They smooth out the emotional rough edges common during menopause and give us some much-needed time to be quiet. Yoga poses, such as twists and backbends,

> Yoga addresses the emotional challenges as well as the physical. When you practice yoga, you learn to slow down your mind and begin to process negative emotions rather than letting them fester.
> —Larry Payne, Ph.D., Richard Usatine, M.D., *Yoga Rx*

Supported Deep Relaxation Pose, also known as Corpse Pose (Savasana): The pause that refreshes during "the pause."

improve the functioning of the adrenals, helping them to increase the amount of estrogen in the body. These poses also stimulate the kidneys, promoting healthy elimination of metabolic by-products.

No aspect of yoga is more important for women crossing the menopausal bridge than to take time every day to practice at least one of yoga's relaxing, restorative poses. Like many women, I have spent my adult life juggling the myriad responsibilities of working outside the home,

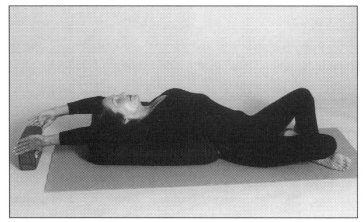

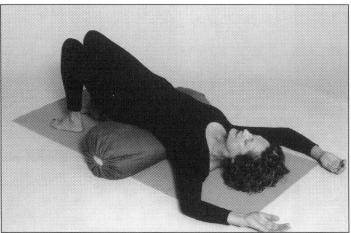

Relaxing on bolsters opens the chest and helps relieve anxiety, irritability and depression.

raising children, caring for animals and doing volunteer work. I was never so grateful to yoga, especially Restorative Yoga, as during these past perimenopausal years. My yoga bolsters, blankets and sticky mat were always in view. I became religious about practicing on a daily basis, no matter how busy I was.

Yoga's Great Rejuvenators—Essential Poses for Crossing the Menopausal Bridge

There are three poses, known in yoga as restorative poses, that I consider essential to practice daily while crossing the menopausal bridge. They are usually referred to as Supported Lying Down Bound Angle Pose, Supported or Elevated Legs Up the Wall Pose and Supported Bridge Pose. It seems fitting to call these three essential poses for the menopausal transition the Goddess Pose, the Great Rejuvenator and the Menopausal Bridge Pose.

The following restorative yoga poses—which include the three essential restorative postures—are recommended for replenishing your adrenal reserves. Equally important, they help calm the mind so that your whole approach to life gradually becomes less hectic and depleting.

Sample Sequence of Poses for Adrenal Exhaustion

Supported Lying Down Bound Angle Pose *(Supta Badha Konasana)* is a healing, nurturing, deeply nourishing pose to practice during the menstrual period and the menopausal transition. It relieves tension and constriction in the abdomen, uterus and vagina. Blood flow

Take advantage of the clarity of vision that is the gift of menopause, and use that gift to let the second half of your life truly be your own.
—Christiane Northrup, M.D., *The Wisdom of Menopause: Creating Physical and Emotional Health and Healing During the Change*

is directed into the pelvis, bathing the reproductive organs and glands and helping to balance hormone function. The centering, balancing effect of this pose helps reduce mood swings and depression. Supported Lying Down Bound Angle Pose is also known for reducing fatigue. For women who suffer from insomnia during menopause, practicing this pose will help you fall asleep at night and recover from lack of sleep during the day. It will also allow the body to relax and open to better breathing. It also helps relieve headaches. It is recommended for digestive problems because of the positive effect on the liver and stomach.

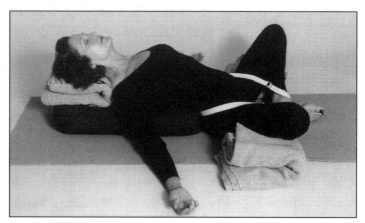

Supported Lying Down Bound Angle Pose, or the Goddess Pose, is essential for crossing the menopausal bridge.

Supported Deep Relaxation Pose *(Savasana)* is part of this series. When you straighten your legs in Supported Lying Down Bound Angle Pose, your body naturally becomes this pose.

Supported Legs Up the Wall Pose *(Viparita Karani,* which means "Inverted Lake") is practiced with the legs up the wall and pelvis elevated on a bolster or folded

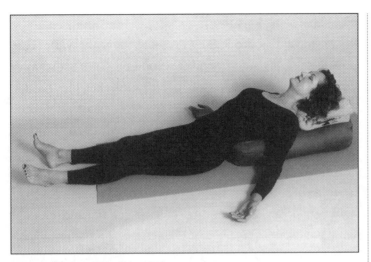

Supported Deep Relaxation Pose.

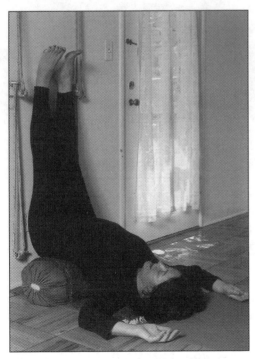

Supported Legs Up the Wall Pose—yoga's "great rejuvenator."

blankets. If the legs tire in the straight position, bend the knees and cross the legs, with knees near the wall. This pose stimulates baroreceptors (blood pressure sensors) in the neck and upper chest, triggering reflexes that reduce nerve input to the adrenal glands, slow heart rate, slow brain waves, relax blood vessels, and reduce the amount of norepinephrine circulating in the bloodstream.

Supported Child's Pose *(Adho Mulcha Virasana)*. It is relaxing to practice Supported Child's Pose in between poses that require you to get up and change your position.

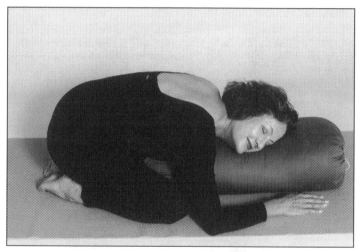

Supported Child's Pose.

Supported Bridge Pose *(Setu Bandha Sarvangasana)* incorporates a bolster or long, folded blankets for support. This pose also stimulates the baroreceptors, so it has many of the same effects as Supported Legs Up the Wall Pose. It relieves tension in the chest and front body and prepares the lungs for breathing practice.

Deep Relaxation Pose *(Savasana)* is practiced with normal inhalations and long, slow exhalations. This

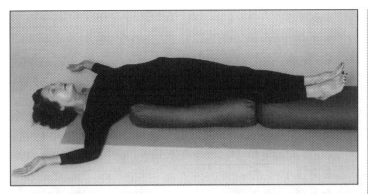

The Menopausal Bridge Pose.

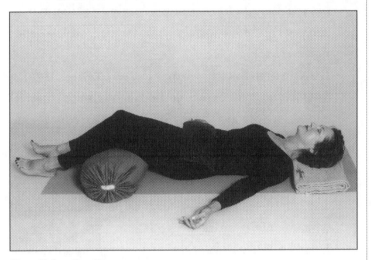

Deep Relaxation Pose.

pose allows complete relaxation in a neutral position. Emphasis on exhalation slows the heart and calms the mind. End your practice with *Savasana*—lying on your back, bolster under knees.

Benefits of Yoga on the Endocrine System

According to B.K.S. Iyengar and doctors who have studied yoga, yoga postures and breathing practices have a beneficial effect on the endocrine system and, if

The role of women in spiritual traditions has often been secondary. Today in America, women are playing essential roles in the evolution of yoga as practitioners, teachers, writers, philosophers and entrepreneurs. Thanks in part to the influence of Geeta Iyengar, we are learning to adapt yoga to our needs, so we can use asanas to help us through each stage of life—menstruation through menopause— with grace, equanimity and self-understanding.

—Patricia Walden,
Yoga Journal,
Sept/Oct '00

practiced regularly, can improve the health of the whole body. Keeping in mind that all menopausal symptoms are related, and that yoga postures act on the whole body, the following yoga poses are especially noted for their beneficial effect on the endocrine system:

- **Backbends:** stimulate thyroid and adrenals; improve circulation in pancreas; relieve pelvic congestion, which benefits ovaries.

- **Bound Angle Pose *(Baddha Konasana)* and Supported Lying Down Bound Angle Pose:** stimulate adrenals and relieve pelvic congestion, which benefits ovaries.

- **Downward-Facing Dog Pose *(Adho Mukha Svanasana):*** tones whole body, thus impacting all endocrine glands; eases hot flashes; reduces the "heavy-headed" feeling associated with menopause.

- **Headstand *(Sirsasana)*:** stimulates pituitary; improves circulation in thyroid; massages the adrenals; stimulates pancreas; relieves pelvic congestion, which benefits ovaries.

- **Head-to-Knee Pose *(Janu Sirsasana)*:** improves circulation in pituitary.

- **Plow Pose *(Halasana)*:** improves circulation in pituitary; provides nourishment (blood) to thyroid; improves circulation in the pancreas and adrenals; stimulates hypothalamus; relieves pelvic congestion, which benefits ovaries.

- **Seated Forward Bend Pose *(Paschimottanasana)*:** improves circulation in pancreas and adrenals; quiets the mind.

- **Seated Cross-Legged Poses:** increase blood flow to adrenals and ovaries.

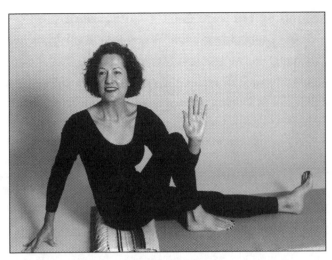

Seated Twist. **Marichyasana III** *front view.*

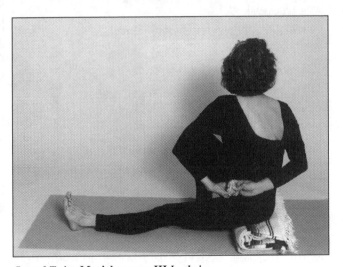

Seated Twist. **Marichyasana III** *backview.*

- **Seated Twist:** replenishes and stimulates adrenals and tones and massages the abdominal organs.
- **Shoulderstand** *(Sarvangasana)*: compresses and massages thyroid and parathyroid; improves circulation in pituitary gland; stimulates pancreas; relieves pelvic congestion, which benefits ovaries.

• **Standing Forward Bend** *(Uttanasana)***:** stimulates all the endocrine glands. When you allow your head to hang below the level of your heart, the pituitary gland, which controls the changes in hormone level that occur during menopause, is stimulated. It also quiets the mind and calms the nervous system.

Factors that Lead to Adrenal Gland Fatigue and Exhaustion

- Chronic illness
- Chronic or severe allergies
- Depression
- Environmental pollution (chronic exposure to industrial or other toxins)
- Excessive amounts of coffee, sugar, salt and other stimulants
- Excessive exercise
- Inadequate sleep
- Light-cycle disruption (inadequate exposure to natural light—e.g., shift work)
- Overwork—physical and mental
- Surgery
- Unhealed trauma or injury

NOTE: The liver is also highly involved in hormone metabolism and benefits greatly from nutritional support and a body-cleansing program.

Key Poses for Adrenal Exhaustion and Fatigue

See chapter 8, "Yoga and the Wisdom of Menopause Practice Guide," for instructions.

Note: All the Essential Restorative Yoga Poses for Crossing the Menopausal Bridge are recommended for adrenal exhaustion. The Restorative Poses listed here can be safely practiced on their own. For example, if you are tired, practice Supported Legs Up the Wall Pose or Supported Lying Down Bound Angle Pose for 10 minutes. If you have 20 minutes, practice both or stay in one pose longer. Do not be in a hurry. Select only the number of poses you can do without feeling rushed.

Pose	Suggested Time
Supported Deep Relaxation Pose	10 minutes
Supported Lying Down Bound Angle Pose	10 minutes
Supported Legs Up the Wall Pose	10 minutes
Supported Bridge Pose	5 to 10 minutes
Deep Relaxation Pose with Bolster Under Legs, Sandbag Across Abdomen	5 to 10 minutes
Additional poses	according to ability
Shoulderstand with Chair	5 minutes
Supported Half Plow Pose	3 to 5 minutes
Other Inverted Poses	according to ability
Rope Headstand	according to ability

The poses listed for balancing your hormones are also helpful for relieving fatigue.

Julie Lawrence, age 55

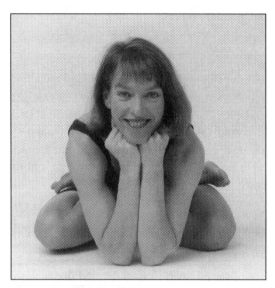

Lotus Posture (**Padmasana**).

First Find Rest

I was desperate. After practicing yoga for almost thirty years I was battling the insomnia demon, and the demon seemed to be winning.

I didn't realize two things. First, my practice of Iyengar yoga had indeed helped to keep most other menopausal symptoms at bay. Second, the effects of the insomnia were cumulative. I had not been sleeping well for three or four years. I wasn't fifty yet, so it couldn't be menopause . . . or could it? I switched health care practitioners when told I was too young (at forty-eight) to be going through menopause. All I knew for sure was that I was exhausted.

My yoga practice had begun to change. I was used to doing a vigorous practice, but my body was yearning for inversions and restorative poses. At one level, my ego rebelled. I did not want to slow down. It meant I was getting old. Yet, on a deeper level, it seemed my heart really heard Geeta Iyengar's advice, "First find rest." I was beginning to realize that maybe I was maturing in my practice . . . and in my life.

I have always marveled at how little yoga it takes to make a difference. My practice began to change, and I found a new appreciation and respect for the power of yoga. It was as though I had been taking it for granted. My evolving practice (which eventually consisted mostly of inversions and restoratives) humbled me and made me more patient with others who also were navigating this journey called menopause. I began to simplify my life in order to conserve energy. The poses I did were simple, deep and delicious.

At the Women's Intensive in Pune, India, in 1997, Geeta instructed us that during menopause we were to, "Stretch well in simple poses." This felt . . . oh, so wise. Yet, even with these changes in my practice, I went to bed each evening fearful that I would wake up in the middle of the night and not be able to go back to sleep. Sometimes I got tense and exhausted just imagining it. The mind can be our worst enemy . . . or our best friend.

I knew the poses to do for insomnia, but there was a part of yoga wisdom that I was neglecting—

that is, the breath. I began doing a relaxation breathing technique three times a day that focused on the power of the exhalation—the releasing, surrendering, accepting aspects of the breath.

Yoga teaches that the mind is the most difficult monkey to train. I began to learn to relax my mind by focusing on the breath, simply the breath. I began to let my mind focus on the quiet beneath my thoughts. I began to move toward my core and eventually feel comfortable there.

Yoga teaches us to be present with whatever is going on. It teaches us to listen and to trust what our body tells us. The body doesn't lie, but we have to be willing to slow down, listen and make decisions about our life based on what we understand to be true.

Yoga brought me home to myself, to feel what my heart wanted and to accept that I needed to slow down and look at my life. With this realization came the split-second decision to take a four-month sabbatical from teaching. This was a huge, frightening stretch for me: Who was I if not a yoga teacher? But it was the best thing I ever did.

Those four months became a period of deep rest. I read, cooked, gardened, spent time with my husband, practiced yoga and came home to myself. The sleep debt was slowly evaporating. I returned to my teaching refreshed and enthused.

During my worst symptoms, no one ever told me that it wouldn't always be like this. Margaret Mead was right—there is such a thing as "postmenopausal zest!" It seems to come from a place of deep authenticity. Sometimes the struggle is exactly what we need to become more fully who we are.

Julie Lawrence, a certified Iyengar yoga instructor and director of the Julie Lawrence Yoga Center in Portland, Oregon, has taught throughout the United States and worldwide since 1976. She has studied in India many times with internationally acclaimed yoga teachers B.K.S. Iyengar and his daughter, Dr. Geeta Iyengar. She lives in Portland, Oregon, with her husband and best friend, Michael Wells.

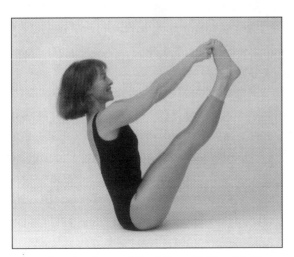

Upward-Facing Forward Bend Pose (**Urdhva Mukha Paschimottanasana**).

Linda DiCarlo, age 55

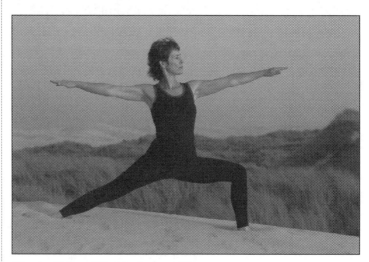

Warrior II Pose (**Virabhadrasana II**).

Compared to my younger years, I now practice with more intelligence and wisdom

Iyengar yoga has been a guiding light in my life since 1986—when it revolutionized my ten-year practice of hatha yoga. Now that I am fifty-five and perimenopausal, it still serves me well. With my teachers' guidance, I have expanded my knowledge and understanding to cultivate sequences based on my energy level, mind-set and emotional nature. I respect the occasional day or two when fatigue sets in and a restorative sequence is more appropriate for me. I have learned the value of supported back-bends to uplift my spirit when I feel flat, and I have grown to appreciate the grounding effect of an inversion practice more than ever before.

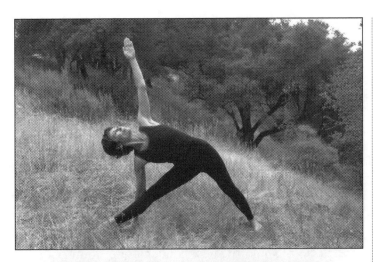

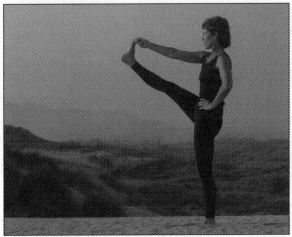

I find myself more strongly drawn to pranayama (regulation of the breath) and dyhana (meditation) and seek the wisdom and solitude promised by diligent pursuit. The vrttis (fluctuations in mind) seem to swirl more with this change of life, and a sitting practice is one of the most treasured parts of my routine now. It is much easier to take the time required, and the rewards are profound and sacred.

In my classes I teach many women who are in their forties and fifties. At this age, hip-opening sequences and poses that keep the thoracic spine supple are imperative. I see these women cultivating their own home practices as they learn the value of steady effort. Some are reluctant to try challenging poses, but with time their confidence grows, they see their classmates going for it and then they are willing to try. Those who persist find they can accomplish more than they initially expected. Some of these students are doing more now than when they were younger. They, too, are learning the value of the tool of yoga for improving the quality of their lives. There is a change that occurs as feelings of respect and reverence come into their hearts. There is an appreciation for the teachings, and an indication that they, too, treasure this ancient centering art.

Linda DiCarlo is an intermediate junior Iyengar yoga instructor and has been teaching yoga since 1978. She enjoys challenging her students and inspiring them to move more deeply into their yoga practice. She lives in Westlake Village, California, teaches classes, workshops and retreats to an eager group of students there and continues to study on a regular basis with her teachers, Patricia Walden and Manouso Manos.

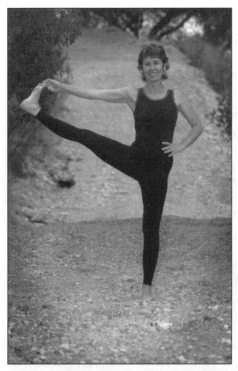

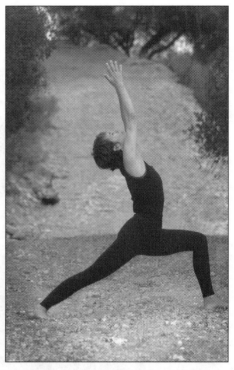

Yoga's balance poses are invigorating and keep your bones strong.

By taking the head back in *Warrior Pose I*, the neck is extended and the thyroid and parathyroid glands are massaged.

Interview with Patricia Walden, age 56

This Is Not the Time to Take On More Things

Patricia Walden is familiar to many through her award-winning yoga videos. She is an expert on yoga for women and created the yoga sequences found in *The Woman's Book of Yoga and Health: A Lifelong Guide to Wellness,* by Linda Sparrowe. Patricia's teaching combines the methodical approach of the Iyengar method with her deep personal experience of the asanas. She directs the B.K.S. Iyengar Yoga Center of Greater Boston and trains teachers throughout the world.

Patricia, what was it like for you, going through menopause? What do you think is most important for women to know about yoga during this stage of their life?

Perimenopause was very interesting for me. I started going into perimenopause around age forty-seven but did not realize what it was. I was keeping a very busy schedule, teaching eight classes a week at my yoga center and traveling a lot. I started getting really tired, adrenally exhausted, but I had no idea it was perimenopause. This was during the summer, and I decided to change my schedule for the coming winter. I gave up five classes and began to travel less. I decided to take a sort of winter sabbatical.

After a while I began to realize I was going through menopause. It was one of these interesting situations where I realized my unconscious was helping me prepare for this period.

It took me awhile to accept what was happening—for example, to accept that it's okay if you're tired, it's okay to back off. I had every possible symptom—hot flashes, insomnia, mood swings. I felt angry, sad. It was a time that my life was turned completely upside down. Interestingly, it was also a time that I felt mentally creative and inspired. But my physiological body could not meet the challenge. I sensed that if I did not pull back I would exhaust myself in a very profound way. So I pulled back for about two years.

How did all of this affect your own yoga practice?

Before all of these symptoms began I had had a very strong practice. But now I had to adjust my practice to suit my needs.

Backbends have always been my favorite poses, but now active backbends put me in an agitated mood. There was a period where Sirsasana (Headstand) did not work. Poses that required exertion and muscular effort did not suit me. But supported *Uttanasana,* (Standing Forward Bend with the head supported) and supported *Adho Mukha Svanasana* (Downward-Facing Dog Pose hanging from a rope or with the head supported on a bolster) felt very good.

Resting your head on a bolster helps cool and energize the brain and relaxes the cranial bones. Circulation is increased to the chest. Supported *Prasaritta Padotanasana* (Widespread Forward Bend) refreshes the brain and soothes the adrenals.

These are all-important poses during menopause. Other seated, supported poses also had a soothing, calming effect.

I really learned how to use my practice to help my nervous system and the changes in my physiological body. There were some days that I felt shaky. I began to be more sensitive to which poses made me shakier and which poses had a soothing effect.

In my practice I emphasized lying on cross bolsters. I experimented and placed the bolsters different ways. As you lie back over the bolster, with your spine and chest supported and your head on the floor, your circulation is increased through the adrenals, thyroid and the kidneys. These poses are very important during menopause because the adrenals take over some of the work of the ovaries. Lying on bolsters in various positions opens the chest, helps you breathe deeply and serves as an antidote to depression.

I placed the bolsters a couple of different ways. How a bolster is placed has a specific effect on your body. How you place your body on the bolsters is also important. There should be no strain in your neck. If you feel discomfort in your back, the feet can be raised on a block or other height. Your chest should be supported at the apex of the pose so that it expands and opens.

In your experience, what are the most important poses for menopause?

Viparita Dandasana (Inverted Staff Pose—a supported backbend practiced lying back over a chair) is a tonic for the nerves and brings a feeling of joy. *Niralamba Sarvangasana* (Supported Shoulderstand—a modification of Shoulderstand with the top of the head to the wall and the toes resting on the wall) is so good for keeping our reproductive organs healthy. Regular practice of this inverted pose may help balance the nervous and endocrine systems.

I would say that the three most important poses during menopause are *Setu Bandha Sarvangasana* (Supported Bridge Pose), Supported *Ardha Halasana* (Half Plow Pose) and lying on cross bolsters with straight legs. The supported variation of *Halasana* quiets the sympathetic nervous system so the brain feels empty and deeply relaxed. I am prone to depression, and these poses recharged my adrenals and were an antidote to depression.

How you practice the poses is as important as which poses you do. Incorrect practice of these poses can leave one feeling more irritated. I've personally had the experience that certain forward bends can bring on a hot flash. When the head position is incorrect, and the neck and shoulders are not released, these poses can create heat in the body. If the head position is correct, then the pose has a cooling effect.

On certain days in a woman's cycle, passive, supported poses help to energize and to integrate. As I mentioned earlier, active poses may cause agitation. In forward bends, small adjustments make a big difference in menopause.

When going through menopause it's important to differentiate between cooling poses and heating poses. During this time we want to focus on cooling poses. Unsupported Headstand created too much heat for me. So on certain days, I practiced a lot of rope *Sirsasana* (Headstand in ropes).

Supported Sirsasana (supported Headstand) works more on the organic body. You are not exerting yourself and holding yourself up with muscular effort.

However, one also has to consider the psychological body, and every practitioner has to determine what practice is most beneficial. Before menopause I had had an active practice, and there were times that I missed this. So on some good days, it was empowering to do active poses. I felt physically tired afterwards but psychologically happy. Having been depressed, I know what I need to keep my emotional body happy. Also, this is a time when you may mourn your youth, and it was empowering to practice strong poses.

This also is a time of reflection and great sensitivity. My practice from outside may look the same, but my experience from inside is unfolding. Working with the natural process of menopause, I found balance. There is a natural pull inwards during menopause. Now my practice has deeper meaning. My meditation and *pranayama* practice has deepened so profoundly these last five years.

What is the most important point you would like women to understand?

If I were to drive home one point to women during this time it would be: Do not take on more stuff. This is a time for you. Our identity is linked so much to how much we do. This is a time to really see who you are in a deeper sense, a time to look at your essence and not just your accomplishments. So often, if we are not doing one hundred things, we feel inadequate. We have to understand deeply that our identity is not what we can do.

Those first perimenopausal years were really humbling. But after that comes a fabulous time when we ripen spiritually. I feel better now than I ever have before.

3 Yoga for Pelvic Health During Perimenopause and Menopause

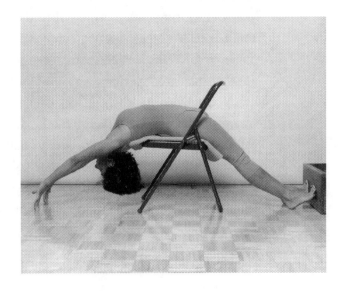

Women's mysteries are of the body and the psyche. A woman may go through the physical experiences that comprise the blood mysteries but miss the soul dimension of being a woman entirely.

—JEAN SHINODA BOLEN, M.D.,
CROSSING TO AVALON: A WOMAN'S MIDLIFE PILGRIMAGE

Yoga's Healing Effect on the Uterus and Ovaries

Many women experience problems with their pelvic organs during perimenopause. In this chapter, we will look at key yoga poses known for supporting pelvic health and alleviating commom symptoms, ranging from heavy bleeding to uterine fibroids to urinary incontinence. Another frequent problem during the perimenopausal years is premenstrual tension resulting from delayed menstrual periods. Upside-Down Bow Pose and Lying Back Over a Chair, Backbender or Bolsters—where the pelvis opens, and the adrenal glands are activated to produce estrogen—may help regulate the menstrual cycle. Backbends such as the Supported Bridge Pose have a powerful physiological effect. They stimulate the ovaries and fallopian tubes, nourish the nervous system and increase the efficiency of the glandular system.

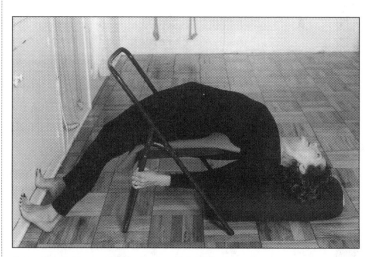

Lying Back Over a Chair (Inverted Staff Pose) relieves menstrual discomfort and helps treat menopausal symptoms.

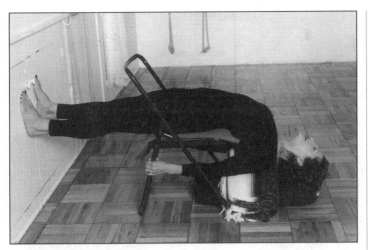

Gentle variation of Lying Back Over a Chair.

Because the uterus is the ark of menopause and the focus of the change, we need to recognize that its evolution into non-bleeding affects our entire feminine body and being, and our entire body and being affect it during this process.
—Farida Sharan, *Creative Menopause*

Women who are beginning yoga during or after menopause can modify the more advanced positions illustrated. Seek the advice of an experienced teacher who can show you how to adjust props so that your neck and back are truly comfortable. Women cannot afford to neglect these tremendously healing and beneficial back-bends during the menopausal years.

Yoga for Frequent or Irregular Bleeding

Women approaching menopause often get their periods too frequently—sometimes as often as two or three times a month. Their menstrual cycles become erratic and may shorten. Conversely, the decrease in ovulation and hormonal output that occurs during perimenopause may contribute to irregular and longer bleeding in many women. A one-week to ten-day menstrual period is not unusual, and some women may bleed through the entire month and longer. This blood loss can be debilitating, because it can lead to anemia. When actual

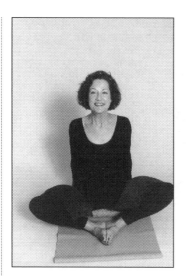
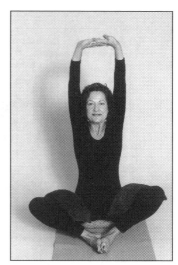

Seated Bound Angle Pose (**Baddha Konasana**) *strengthens the bladder and uterus and eases perimenopausal symptoms.*

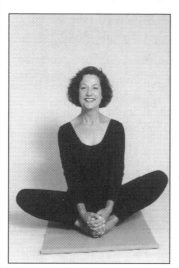
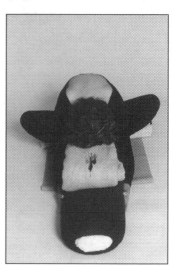

menopause and cessation of periods approaches, the irregular menstrual pattern reverses, with the periods becoming farther apart and lighter.

Many other factors—including emotional stress, inadequate nutrition, excessive alcohol intake, cigarette

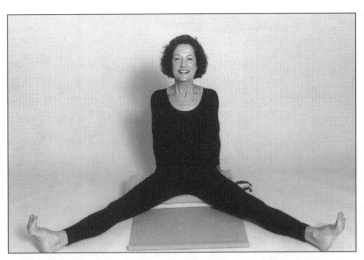

Seated Wide Angle Pose (**Upavista Konasana**) *increases circulation in the pelvic region and helps lift and tone your uterus.*

smoking and environmental conditions—can exacerbate bleeding problems and make women more susceptible to heavy, irregular bleeding.

To relieve bleeding between normal periods, I recommend that women practice healing postures such as Seated Wide Angle Pose, Seated and Lying Down Supported Bound Angle Poses and inverted poses. Inverted poses and backbends stimulate the endocrine glands and improve their functioning. An endocrine disorder can also be improved by yoga postures and breathing practices *(pranayama)*, which involve prolonging and restraining the breath and help regulate hormonal levels in the blood.

Note: Many environmental factors and nutritional deficiencies can worsen bleeding problems. While most cases of irregular heavy bleeding are due to fluctuating hormonal levels as your body moves through menopause, other medical problems can cause heavy bleeding. Any serious bleeding problem should be evaluated by your doctor.

This is what you have to remember: that when the flow is between the normal periods, you have to do the healing asanas such as *Upavistha Konosana* (Seated Wide Angle Pose), *Baddha Konasana* (Bound Angle Pose) and Inversions. Sitting and forward extensions also help but in these asanas you have to learn to lift up the pelvic organs.

—B.K.S. Iyengar

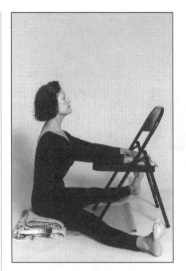

A chair helps open the chest and lengthen the spine.

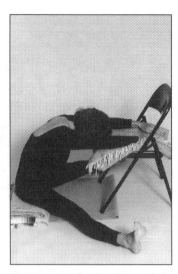

Resting your forehead on a chair helps your brain to relax.

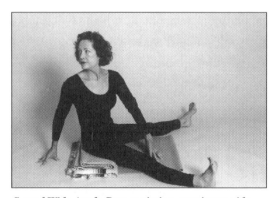

Seated Wide Angle Pose variation, turning to side.

Cautions About Upside-Down (Inverted) Poses When Bleeding

Many of my students and readers ask whether they should completely avoid inverted (upside-down) poses while they are menstruating. As a rule, inverted poses should not be practiced during menstruation. Women who experience irregular bleeding are also generally advised not to practice inverted poses when they are bleeding.

One of my readers put into writing a question I am frequently asked about inverted poses:

I am a yoga student and practice regularly. I am perimenopausal, and my periods are becoming frequent and irregular. I would like to know if these periods should be treated as "normal" in the sense that I should not do inversions. Sometimes they come every couple of weeks and last five or six days with normal bleeding. Sometimes they can last for ten to twelve days with a very heavy flow. I suffer no pain or PMS. I rarely have hot flashes or trouble sleeping. I am healthy. My gynecologist says this a natural progression, but she doesn't have any knowledge of yoga. Do you know if I should refrain from inverting during both types of periods?

I consulted several woman teachers who are experts in women's health and yoga. Based on my own experience as well, I would concur with their advice: Do *not* practice any inversions when spotting. Instead, practice supported backbends and supported lying down poses such as Lying Down Bound Angle Pose. When you are not bleeding, you can practice many inversions.

In my previous book, *The New Yoga for People Over 50,* in the chapter on *Yoga and Menopause,* I briefly discuss the situation where women get their periods too frequently—sometimes as often as two or three times a month. According to B.K.S. Iyengar, "This 'in-between-period bleeding' is not the same as menstrual bleeding. The in-between bleeding may be caused by irritation

Practice the *Supta* cycle (lying down poses) with a minimum of disturbance, to achieve a deep rest and relaxation from the poses. Allow your abdomen, uterus and ovaries to remain soft and let your groin open, and descend. Broaden and soften your pelvis. Properly resting in these poses is more helpful than lying in bed.

—Jeanne Marie Derrick, *Yoga for Menstruation*

within the uterus. For example, if after seven days of a regular period the flow has decreased, the yoga practice should be adjusted to further decrease bleeding. Exertion poses that stimulate the ovaries may increase the flow and prolong the period."

I advise readers who experience this type of bleeding to seek out the guidance of a knowledgeable teacher. Having said that, I must also mention that not all teachers advise against doing inverted poses during menstruation. Some teachers believe that the choice varies from woman to woman.

Teachers who *do* advise against practicing inversions point out that certain physical problems may result. Until recently, increased risk of endometriosis was considered the most common risk. But since more is known now about this disease, the idea has been repudiated.

There is also a theory that inversions may cause "vascular congestion" in the uterus, resulting in excessive menstrual flow. If this is true, the risk probably applies mainly to experienced practitioners who stay in inverted poses for long periods. In my own practice, I generally take the middle path. Back when I was still having periods, if it was on or toward the last day, and I was longing to leap into a Handstand (Full Arm Balance) for a minute or so, I would spontaneously do so.

Some teachers also point out that philosophically speaking, menstruation is considered to be *apana,* meaning that, energetically, its vitality is downward flowing. The argument against turning your body upside down during menstruation is that this will disturb the natural downward energy flow.

Confusion also arises because there seems to be contradictory advice from certain highly regarded teachers.

Their writings seem to suggest that practicing inversions can alleviate menstrual problems such as heavy flow and irregular periods. However, it is not clear in these writings whether inversions should only be practiced when a woman is not bleeding or, if working under the guidance of a knowledgeable teacher, there are exceptions to the "no inversions during menstruation rule."

To be on the safe side, it makes sense to me to *avoid* practicing inverted poses when you are spotting or bleeding.

Upside-Down Poses After the Menstrual Period

The classic yoga texts, *Light on Yoga* by B.K.S. Iyengar and *Yoga: A Gem for Women* by his daughter,

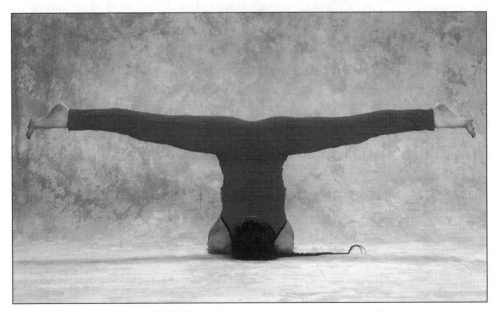

Ana Forrest in Shoulderstand with feet wide apart (**Upavista Konasana** *in* **Sarvangasana**).

Geeta Iyengar, recommend that Headstand and Shoulderstand be practiced after every menstrual period to ensure inner dryness once bleeding has stopped. Experienced teachers caution women against switching *too* quickly to their usual, more active practice after menstruation. Women who follow the recommended gentle, supported forward bends and restorative practices during the menstrual period, and then resume a routine of more strenuous standing, backbending and balancing poses immediately after, may run the risk of overexerting themselves. Some teachers believe that this may contribute to health problems as one gets older, especially during the perimenopausal years.

It seems wise to consider the yoga practice immediately following one's period as a healing practice. Inverted poses and their variations, practiced *after* bleeding stops, heal the reproductive organs, the organs affected by menopause. B.K.S. Iyengar recommends a long, quiet stay in Headstand or Shoulderstand, without too many variations. Iyengar writes, "Straight asanas keep you cool, calm, quiet; and when that feeling has come, the mind gets subdued."

The long, motionless holding of inversions opens the door to a state of meditation. It is during and after the peaceful practice of inversions that one experiences poise, peace and stillness at a deeper level. A long stay in the poses quiets and strengthens the nervous system, an invaluable gift at all stages of life, but most especially during the menopausal transition.

Inversions and Menstruation

Mary Pullig Schatz, M.D., advises against inverting while menstruating because it may lead to vascular congestion. The uterine veins, which are thin, can stretch and partially collapse, while uterine arteries continue to pump more menstrual blood into the uterus. If inversions cause you to bleed more than usual during your period, you may become weak and feel emotionally less stable.

Yoga to Alleviate Pelvic Congestion, Pelvic Pain and Cramps

Lying Down Bound Angle Pose is considered by many to be one of the most effective poses for both regulating and balancing a woman's menstrual cycle and relieving symptoms associated with menopause. Blood flow is directed to the pelvis, bathing the reproductive organs and glands and helping to balance hormone function. The pose relieves tension and constriction in the abdomen, uterus and vagina. The centering, balancing effect of Lying Down Bound Angle Pose helps reduce mood swings, anxiety and depression. This pose is additionally beneficial for those with high blood pressure, headaches and breathing problems.

All inverted poses, forward bends, Seated Bound Angle Pose (sitting upright with the soles of the feet together), Supported Lying Down Bound Angle Pose, Lying Down Big Toe Pose with Leg Opened Up to Side, and Seated Wide Angle Pose, help reduce pelvic congestion and improve circulation to the pelvic area.

Headstand, Lying Back Over a Chair, Shoulderstand, Plow Pose and seated forward bends have specific influences on the psychoneurohormonal system. These postures help reduce tension and thus help reduce menopausal symptoms.

The poses B.K.S. Iyengar recommends for discomfort related to the menstrual cycle demonstrate his three cardinal principles of therapeutic yoga: spreading (creating space for fresh blood to enter the organ); soaking (providing time and space for fresh blood to bathe and nourish the organ); and squeezing (removing used blood and fluid by pressure). This approach helps alleviate pain related to pelvic congestion.

On a physical level, yoga eases menstrual and menopausal problems by relaxing the nervous system, balancing the endocrine system, increasing the flow of blood and oxygen to the reproductive organs, and strengthening the muscles surrounding those organs.

Psychologically, yoga works to ease stress and promote relaxation. It offers a woman the opportunity to go deep inside and learn about her body from the inside out.

Menstrual Problems and Nutritional Remedies

Women often experience a feeling of heaviness and congestion before and during their period and in the months after their periods have stopped. This is an excellent time to make dietary improvements and to consider a body-cleansing program. Adding fresh fruits and vegetables to your diet will help reduce feelings of heaviness in the abdomen.

One factor in the various contributing causes of menstrual disturbances is excessive estrogen activity, a by-product of disturbed liver function, which in turn is due to poor eating habits. Henry Bieler, M.D., points out in his classic *Food Is Your Best Medicine*, that the duration and amount of menstrual flow is greatly influenced by diet and lifestyle, as are the effects on a woman's body when the menstrual period stops.

Bieler says, "Misled by the idea that the average represents what is 'normal,' many women have been persuaded to accept pathological states of menstrual problems simply because they are so prevalent. However, excessive and heavy menstrual flow, cramping, lower back pain, and pelvic congestion may be indications that the liver is failing as a 'filter'.

"When toxic blood seeks an outlet through the womb via the menstrual function, the resulting inflammation and irritation to the delicate mucous membranes throw the organ into spasms which are registered as pain or cramps (or simply congestion if the toxin is more dilute). . . . Once the flow has started, nature pours out as much toxic material from the blood as possible. . . . What should be a normal flow develops into a hemorrhage, sometimes lasting for days and reducing the woman to a state of anemia. Nervousness, insomnia, headache and distressing fatigue may follow. The kidneys may not be able to sufficiently filter certain diffusible poisons so that a mild-to-severe edema occurs, evidenced by an increase in body weight. The woman who suffers menstrual problems during her menstrual years may

> also have health problems during menopause, when she can no longer discharge toxins through the menstrual blood."

Note to yoga teachers, doctors and other health professionals: Please refer to *A Matter of Health,* by Dr. Krishna Raman, for an in-depth discussion of yogic management of fibroids of the uterus and other gynecological conditions common during perimenopause and menopause. (See Resources.)

Key Poses for Pelvic Health

See chapter 8, "Yoga and the Wisdom of Menopause Practice Guide," for instructions.

Reminder: Do not be in a hurry. Select only the number of poses you can do without feeling rushed. **Time suggested is the minimum time.** Experienced practitioners can stay in poses longer.

Note: These poses are recommended during menstruation and all through your monthly cycle.

Pose	Suggested Time
Supported Lying Down Bound Angle Pose	10 minutes
Seated Bound Angle Pose	2 to 5 minutes
Seated Wide Angle Pose	2 to 5 minutes
Supported Half Moon Pose (If weak and flowing heavily, skip standing poses)	30 seconds, longer if experienced
Lying Back Over a Chair, Backbender or Bolsters	length of time according to comfort—1 to 5 minutes
Lying Down Big Toe Pose with Leg Opened Up to Side, Supported by Bolster	1 minute
Supported Deep Relaxation Pose	5 minutes
To Practice When You Are *Not* Bleeding:	**Suggested Time**
Supported Legs Up the Wall Pose	10 minutes
All inverted poses	according to ability

Poses for Strengthening the Pelvic Floor and Helping Urinary Incontinence:	Suggested Time
Standing and Seated Poses	
Wide Angle Standing Forward Bends	1 minute
Downward-Facing Dog Pose	1 minute
Seated Bound Angle Pose	1 minute
Seated Wide Angle Pose	1 minute
Supported Lying Down Bound Angle Pose	10 minutes
For Experienced Practitioners:	**Suggested Time**
Headstand and Shoulderstand with variations, soles of your feet together or legs wide apart	according to ability
Backbends, both supported and active, practiced with guidance of experienced teacher, can help correct displaced bladder or prolapsed uterus	according to ability
Ask your teacher about the Great Seal Pose (Maha Mudra) practiced in Head to Knee Pose (*Janusirsasana*)	

Practice Kegels, the inner pelvic floor lifting exercise learned in childbirth classes, in daily life. Ask your teacher about *Aswini Mudra* and *Mula Bandha*, the contraction and muscular lifting up of the floor of the pelvis.

Diana Rose Hartmann, age 42

Tossed Over the Bridge into Menopause

My menopause came about in a hurry. I had a hysterectomy when I was forty and lost my ovaries the following year. I was devastated—I had wanted a child.

Before my hysterectomy, I was bleeding twelve days or more per month due to fibroid tumors. I practiced yoga remedies, had acupuncture treatments, took herbs, meditated, prayed and gave up any and every food that might contribute to my fibroids. None of this worked. I had a myomectomy (removal of fibroids) to help me conceive, and tried artificial insemination and ovulation kits—but nothing helped. To make matters worse, my marriage was not going well, sex was painful and I already felt less than womanly because of my infertility.

My hormones took a nosedive after my hysterectomy, but I was too grief-stricken to notice all the effects. I had one or two hot flashes. My breasts became hollow and sagging. I was in denial about losing my uterus, and for months I couldn't even throw away my leftover menstrual pads. It didn't help that my husband and I had separated; two weeks after the loss of my uterus he mentioned divorce.

I began to take yoga classes to help with my grief and depression. The deeper yoga I began doing now incorporated intense backbends and helped me with my grief. On the way home from a particularly good class, I would sob. It was a good cry, the kind that feels as if a weight has been lifted from your shoulders. Other times, it felt as if my entire perception had been changed. I would drive home and the trees would seem brighter, the sky lighter—and I would reconnect with a joy that had been lacking in my life for years.

Because the intense yoga postures helped my emotional state, I pushed myself. I certainly wasn't ready to "find rest." I wanted to prove that I was a woman. I tried to keep my body firm by doing Astanga or power yoga, along with the deeper Iyengar-style yoga. I ignored the persistent pain in my left side, where my ovary was.

Almost a year went by and finally I couldn't take the pain anymore. I was visiting the local emergency room every three months because the pain became so bad that it was necessary for me to take narcotic painkillers. An ultrasound revealed that I had a hemorrhagic cyst that came and went on my left ovary. I continued to do yoga, eat right and work on my novel. I was in too much pain to work outside my home, and the yoga kept me from feeling completely isolated.

I asked my yoga teacher about cysts and yoga, and he said that cysts were one thing that even Iyengar couldn't find a cure for. I thought that perhaps I had adhesions. My gynecologist suggested an exploratory laparoscopic surgery. I agreed. I never thought of "resting." I never thought of taking care of myself, of acknowledging my grief, of letting my body get a little softer or fatter. I kept working to prove to myself (and my estranged husband) that I was a young, attractive woman.

Before the surgery, I tried to prepare myself for the possibility that I might lose my left ovary. I wasn't too worried. Right before I went under anesthesia, my mother—a retired nurse—reassured me that having one ovary was not the same as having no ovaries. When I awoke, however, my mother had the same look of despair on her face that she had had six years ago—right before she told me that my beloved cat had been run over. The doctor had found endometriosis and so had removed not one, but both my ovaries. I was instantly put on a patch, a natural form of estrogen.

Well, there I was—marked with a sticky estrogen patch and tossed over the bridge of menopause at forty-one years of age! I tried to convince my husband that I could be the wife he wanted, even if it meant giving up whatever sense of self I had left. My whole world seemed to fall apart. After this surgery, which was even more of a stress on my body than the hysterectomy, I barely allowed myself six weeks of restorative yoga postures before jumping back into my intermediate class.

Strangely, the poses that had worked for me before the removal of my ovaries now ceased to work. My body had changed, and dramatically so. I enrolled in an intermediate intensive and had a different sort of experience. I was shaky and felt disconnected. I was irked because we weren't doing enough inversions. Backbends didn't seem to do what they used to do. The teacher forbade me to do one of my favorite postures, *Viparita Dandasana* (a backbend), using the wall ropes, because he noticed it was aggravating my nervous system. Even head-stands didn't feel that great anymore.

For some reason, my nerves now craved inward postures. Once I got into *Savasana* (Deep Relaxation Pose), I didn't want to get out of it. And I found comfort practicing a few of the advanced poses at home: *Kurmasana* (Tortoise Pose) and *Yogidrasana* (an advanced pose with the legs crossed behind the head). My ego still wants to do Astanga to keep my body fit, but my inner self won't let me. I can do a few backbends, but if I do too many, too much grief is released.

The day I read Suza's introduction, I realized that by the work of angels I was being told to accept that I was catapulted into menopause, whether I liked it or not. I needed to hear the wisdom of women who were wiser than me, elder women who were crossing over or had already made it to the other side of the bridge. I still feel the impulse to act as a nonmenopausal woman of forty-two. But I have discovered I need to slow down, to use the wonderful tool of yoga in a different way and to really take a pause.

I'm a full-fledged member of menopause. It is not something I need to be ashamed of—it is not the end of my womanhood. It is a time to go inward and redefine myself. It is a time to realize that while

I was not able to bear children in this life, I can still aid in the midwifery of books, which I see as brain-children, little angels in themselves. They can make their way in the world and touch the hearts of fellow human beings just as biological children can.

Diana Rose Hartmann is a writer, editor and yoga teacher. She began her yoga studies twenty years ago. As the years passed, she would lose interest in yoga for a few months, but, she says, "Whenever my life became crazy, or I felt I was losing my center, I knew yoga was there for me and took advantage of it." She has studied many styles of yoga with numerous teachers. For the past several years, she's had the good fortune of studying with Aadil Palkhivala, whom she credits with really helping her understand her body in a deeper way. She's learned that while home practice is important, a good teacher is a necessity.

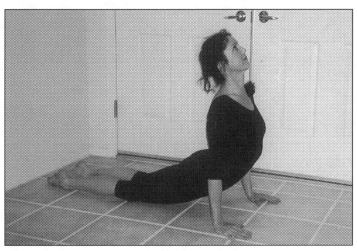

Upward-Facing Dog Pose (Urdhva Mukha Svanasana).

4 The Power of Hot Flashes

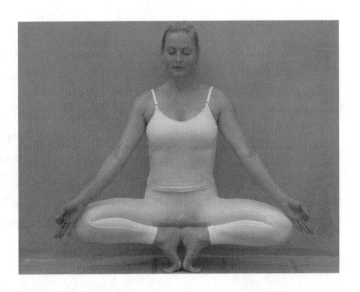

You can use hot flashes as a personal wake-up call:
"Wake up! Something powerful is happening!"
Use this changing time before it passes to access and
study your old behaviors, sweat out what no longer
works—the poisons and toxins you have accumulated
in your lifetime—and to let go of old hatreds and
resentments. The more you use your hot flashes,
the more skillful you become in transforming
energy, and thus your life.

—ANA FORREST, YOGA TEACHER

Hot flashes or flushes—or "power surges," as many women prefer to call them—are the most common symptom of menopause. They fall under a category of physical symptoms known as vasomotor changes and, therefore, are also known as vasomotor flushes. Vasomotor changes are alterations in blood circulation that cause temperature fluctuations. Hot flashes, night sweats, insomnia and, possibly, heart palpitations, are all a result of vasomotor changes.

Hot flashes are the result of sudden changes in the body's "thermostat," the center of the brain that controls temperature regulation. If a woman's hypothalamus perceives that she is too warm, it starts a chain of events designed to cool her down. Blood vessels near the surface of the body begin to dilate so that blood can carry excess heat away from the skin. This produces a red, flushed appearance on the face and neck. Some women also begin to perspire profusely so that the evaporating sweat can cool the body. A sudden increase in pulse rate may also occur. Because of these changes, a cold chill sometimes follows; in fact, a few women experience only the chill.

Some hot flashes, accompanied by drenching perspiration, occur while sleeping. These are referred to as night sweats. Night sweats and hot flashes may interfere with healthy, deep sleep. Menopause itself cannot be blamed for feeling irritable, but inadequate sleep causes fatigue, which does result in irritability. Because hot flashes involve the neuroendocrine system, unresolved stress also tends to increase them.

More than two-thirds of North American women have hot flashes during the menopausal years. Some women experience hot flashes for only a few months, others for several years. A small percentage reports hot flashes for a decade or more. Many yoga teachers and students report that a regular yoga practice can help alleviate these symptoms.

Alternative Theories on Hot Flashes

What if hot flashes—like so much about menopause—have been misunderstood by modern culture? What if hot flashes are a sign of the body's wisdom—a physical, psychological and spiritual process aimed at moving us in the direction of health and wholeness? What if hot flashes are a unique opportunity for self-knowledge and self-awareness, rather than an uncomfortable and embarrassing symptom?

Numerous leaders in the fields of complementary and alternative women's health have been asking exactly these questions. Dr. Joan Borysenko believes that hot flashes represent a rebalancing of energy that can help women burn off stress, rather than add to it. This idea has some basis in Chinese medicine and yoga philosophy. In her exceptional book on the feminine life cycle, *A Woman's Book of Life,* Dr. Borysenko writes:

> *During the perimenopausal years, the Chinese believe that there is an increase in the active, dry, hot element called yang energy. Before thirty-five a woman is more yin (moist, receptive, passive), but during the change of life her yang begins to express itself. She becomes more passionate about ideas, quicker to anger, faster to defend herself and others. As more "hot" yang energy begins to move through the acupuncture*

Ten years ago, at age forty-five, I started to experience strong hot flashes, mood swings, memory loss and depression. My doctor told me that since my father died from having had seven heart attacks, and that I was starting menopause, I should go on Prozac and hormone replacement therapy. Not believing in either remedy, I took up yoga again and found a naturopathic doctor. I felt as if yoga was my medicine. Every day I made sure that I included Headstand and Shoulderstand in my practice, thinking of these two poses as my daily prescription against illness. Most of my menopausal symptoms seemed to disappear.

—Dale Mirmow, yoga teacher

meridians, at first the flow is somewhat jerky as we get accustomed to using new energy. Those jerky manifestations of rising yang give rise to hot flashes.

According to Dr. Borysenko and others, forty-nine different cultural traditions base their medicine on the concept of life-force energy. When we have too much stress, the life-force energy can't flow smoothly through the acupuncture meridians. This can be the result of inadequate nutrition, lack of sleep and exercise, emotional factors, overwork or any number of midlife circumstances converging in ways that are less than ideal.

From the perspective of yoga philosophy, a hot flash represents the release of kundalini (cosmic life-force) energy which "rewires" the nervous system. In this view, the hot flash is a kind of natural stress-release mechanism that discharges trauma and other energies locked in the body over the course of a lifetime. This process chips away at our "character armor" and forces us to address major issues of personal integration.

Hot flashes may also be triggered by certain foods. For information on herbs and foods to manage hot flashes naturally, I highly recommend Susun Weed's, *(New) Menopausal Years: The Wise Woman Way* (see Resources section for her Web site).

Hot Flashes May Be Healthy

Although most women who experience hot flashes seek relief, some researchers believe the increase in the body's surface temperature might serve a useful function. Vickie Noble, author of *Shakti Woman: Feeling Our Fire, Healing Our World,* feels that hot flashes may actually be healthy. She reminds us that a high body temperature kills bacteria. When we attempt to shut down the hot-flash process, we might be interfering with a subtle healing mechanism.

Cooling Yoga Poses for Hot Flashes, Day/Night Sweats and Other Menopausal Symptoms

For centuries, classic inverted postures, especially the Shoulderstand, Plow Pose and Downward-Facing Dog Pose, as well as various relaxing forward bends and restorative poses, have been valued for their cooling, calming effect on the mind and nervous system.

To position all or just the upper portion of the body upside down may greatly reduce the incidence and intensity of hot flashes and night sweats. Over the years, my students, as well as teachers that I've studied with, have told me that inverted poses when practiced on a regular basis are an effective antidote for hot flashes and other common menopausal symptoms. A long stay in

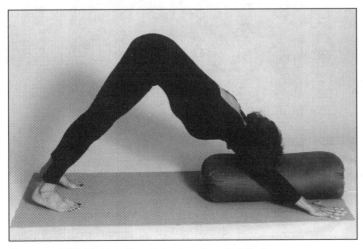

Downward-Facing Dog Pose helps to relieve hot flashes.

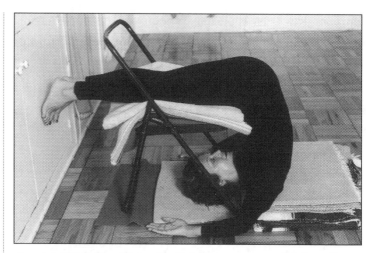

Supported Half Plow Pose calms the nervous system and helps relieve hot flashes.

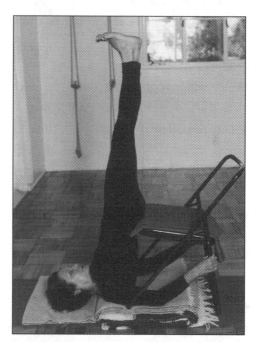

Shoulderstand eases many menopausal symptoms, including hot flashes.

Shoulderstand, or a Shoulderstand variation known as *Niralamba Sarvangasana,* has a particularly quieting effect on the brain and nervous system.

Inverted poses also have a dramatic effect on what physiologists call hemodynamics—the flow of blood to every organ of the body. They have a particularly potent—and measurable—effect on the glands of the endocrine system, including the pineal, pituitary, thyroid, parathyroid, adrenals and hypothalamus. Keep in mind that the endocrine system controls the changes in hormone levels that occur during menopause.

According to psychobiologist and yoga teacher Roger Cole, Ph.D., who has conducted extensive scientific studies on the physiological effects of yoga poses, turning the body upside down also tricks the body into believing that blood pressure has risen, because the receptors that measure blood pressure are all in the neck and chest region. The body then takes immediate steps to lower blood pressure, including relaxing blood vessels and reducing the hormones that cause retention of water and salt. These physiological adjustments may help ease menopausal symptoms.

On a more subtle level, inverted poses affect the flow of *prana*—or life-force energy—in a way that can help counteract hot flashes. Inverted poses draw *prana* inward, toward our vital organs and the body's core, and *away* from the surface (the skin). According to some theories, during hot flashes, *prana* is flowing outward from the body's center, heating the skin.

Supported Legs Up the Wall Pose, Supported Shoulderstand, the Shoulderstand variation known as *Niralamba Sarvangasana*, Supported Half Plow Pose *(Ardha Halasana)* and Downward-Facing Dog Pose are all inverted postures recommended by yoga practitioners as helpful in mitigating the effects of hot flashes.

Yoga is not about the body or about the mind. It is about the synthesis of body and mind, and the transformed self that is the result. It is an adventure in human potential, in going beyond the spirit identity that neither body alone nor mind alone provides, in discovering a new kind of energy and life.
—Dona Holleman and Orit Sen-Gupta, *Dancing the Body Of Light: The Future of Yoga*

For Experienced Practitioners:
Niralamba Sarvangasana

According to Geeta Iyengar, daughter of B.K.S. Iyengar and author of *Yoga: A Gem for Women,* a Shoulderstand variation known as *Niralamba Sarvangasana* is more effective for hot flashes than even *Sarvangasana* on the chair. Although the classic *Niralamba Sarvangasana,* when practiced without support, is more challenging than Shoulderstand, the supported variation developed by B.K.S. Iyengar makes this pose possible for experienced students who are familiar with Shoulderstand and practice it regularly. Experienced students working with the guidance of a teacher can practice supported *Niralamba Sarvangasana* instead of, or in addition to, classical *Salamba Sarvangasana.*

The benefits of *Niralamba Sarvangasana* are a boon to women during menopause, especially when practiced in the evening after an active day, or when practiced to recover from an illness. This pose is highly recommended for keeping the reproductive organs healthy. Regular practice of *Niralamba Sarvangasana* may also help remedy dysfunction or imbalance in the central nervous, reproductive and endocrine systems. Many consider it a boost for womankind!

Caution: I do not recommend this pose until you are completely familiar with and secure practicing Shoulderstand with a chair. I am including it here to expand your knowledge of the potential yoga holds for helping women with common symptoms like hot flashes.

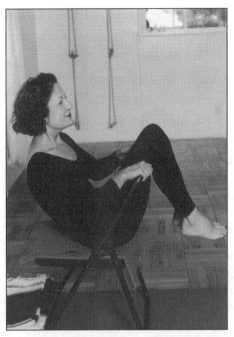

Preparation for Shoulderstand and variations such as **Niralamba Sarvangasana.**

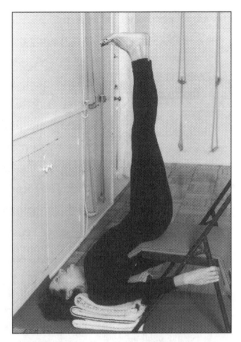

Shoulderstand with chair variation that leads into **Niralamba Sarvangasana.**

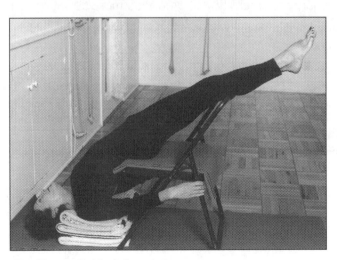

Shoulderstand with chair variation.

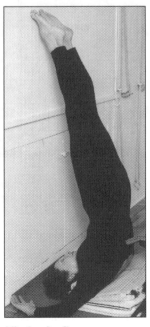

Niralamba Sarvangasana.

Our physical manifestation is a doorway to the deeper inward journey of spiritual awakening. The purpose of life is to recognize our own perfection and divinity, and yoga offers a path to that realization. . . . I look at hot flashes as a gift. I think they are the body's natural response to the changes that are happening—not to be stopped, altered or managed by medication or any other artificial means.

—Susan Winter Ward, yoga teacher

Lying Back Over a Chair or Backbender *(Viparita Dandasana)* and Supported Bridge Pose are some of the other poses associated with cooling hot flashes.

In contrast, several longtime yoga practitioners interviewed for this book reported that classic Headstand, requiring strength and exertion, did not work for them during menopause—or at least not during certain phases of their menopause. However, Rope Headstand (Hanging Upside Down in Yoga Wall Ropes) and other restful, supported variations of both Headstand and Shoulderstand had a positive, cooling and calming effect (see chapter 8).

Creative Menopause

In her illuminating book on women's health and spirituality, *Creative Menopause*, Farida Sharan describes her experience with hot flashes: "Toward the fourth month the releases increased in purity, beauty and intensity. As I grounded more deeply in my being, I began to perceive the reality of my life around me in a different way. My martyr persona was dissolving. I could no longer do things the way I always had. I saw more deeply. It was as though I read people's minds and motives and looked at my life and realized I would have to change."

Menopause and Kundalini—The Kundalini Energy-Hot Flash Connection

Susun Weed believes that hot flashes are "kundalini training sessions," not a pathological condition. They are a powerful rite of passage and a transformative part of a woman's life. In her view, hot flashes are "power surges" and the "change" is the intense spiritual journey of the crone.

As a longtime student of yoga, Susun Weed was struck by the many similarities between menopausal symptoms and the well-known esoteric goal of awakening the kundalini. She writes:

Kundalini is the root of all spiritual experience . . . Kundalini is a special kind of energy known in many cultures, including Tibetan, Indian, Sumerian, Chinese, Irish, Aztec and Greek. Kundalini is said to be hot, fast, powerful and large. It exists within the earth, within all life, and within each person. Psychoanalyst Carl G. Jung called kundalini "anima." Kundalini is usually represented as a serpent coiled at the base of the spine, but women's mystery stories locate it in the uterus—or the area where the uterus was, if a hysterectomy has occurred. During both puberty and menopause, a woman's kundalini is difficult to control and may cause a great number of symptoms.

East Indian yogis spend lifetimes learning to activate, or wake up, their kundalini. This is also called "achieving enlightenment." When they succeed, a surge of super-heated energy goes up the spine, throughout the nerves, dilating blood vessels, and fueling itself with hormones. As kundalini continues to travel up the spine, it changes the functioning of the endocrine, cardiovascular and nervous systems. Not just in yogis, but in any woman who allows herself to become aware of it. Menopause is a kind of enlightenment. Hot flashes are kundalini training sessions.

Hot Flash Studies

Stress intensifies almost every symptom of menopause, including hot flashes. Reducing stress by making lifestyle and behavioral changes, and making yoga a regular part of your life, can have a positive effect on managing hot flashes.

A variety of studies and many individual women report good results by practicing slow, deep breathing when a hot flash is starting. In one study on the effect of breathing and other yoga-based stress reduction techniques, women who practiced "paced respiration" had 40 percent fewer hot flashes than the rest of the women in the study group. It makes sense, when you feel a flash coming on, to be aware of your breathing and practice slow, calm inhalations and exhalations.

Researchers at the School of Medicine at Wayne State University studied thirty-three women with frequent hot flashes and measured their responses to deep breathing, muscle relaxation and brain-wave biofeedback. Deep breathing was associated with a significant reduction in the frequency of hot flashes, while the other two techniques had no effect. The authors speculate that deep breathing somehow works to alter the sympathetic nervous system activity that gives rise to hot flashes.

Good Reading

The Menopausal Years: The Wise Woman Way, by Susun S. Weed

Creative Menopause, by Farida Sharan

The Wisdom of Menopause, by Christiane Northrup, M.D.

A Woman's Book of Life, by Joan Borysenko, Ph.D.

Key Poses to Ease Hot Flashes

See chapter 8, "Yoga and the Wisdom of Menopause Practice Guide," for instructions.

Reminder: Do not be in a hurry. Select only the number of poses you can do without feeling rushed. **Time suggested is the minimum time.** Experienced practitioners can stay in poses longer. Supporting the head increases the benefits.

Pose	Suggested Time
Seated Bound Angle Pose	1 to 5 minutes
Seated Wide Angle Pose	1 to 5 minutes
Supported Standing Forward Bend Pose	1 minute
Wide Angle Standing Forward Bend with Head Supported	1 to 5 minutes
Downward-Facing Dog Pose	1 minute
Supported Shoulderstand	5 minutes
Niralamba Sarvangasana (variation of Shoulderstand)	5 minutes
Supported Half Plow Pose	3 to 5 minutes
Supported Bridge Pose	5 to 10 minutes
Supported Lying Down Bound Angle Pose	10 minutes
Supported Legs Up the Wall Pose	10 minutes
Deep Relaxation Pose	10 minutes

Interview with Susan Winter Ward, age 58

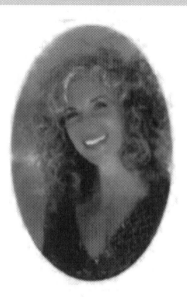

Embracing Menopause:
A Path to Peace and Power

You're fifty-eight. Are you postmenopausal? Do you still have hot flashes or other symptoms?

It's been several years since I've had a period, but I still have hot flashes. The other day I spoke to a woman who has had them for twenty-five years. If they never stop that's okay with me. I look at hot flashes as a gift. I think they are the body's natural response to changes that are happening—not something to be stopped, altered or managed by medication or any other artificial means. They can be uncomfortable at times, but they are also a gift. And here in Colorado, they come in handy at the ski lift.

Sometimes women ask, "How do you know it's a hot flash?"

This is what I tell women who are not sure if it's a hot flash: If you are standing naked in front of the freezer with the door open at 2 A.M.—it's a hot flash!

Forty-five million American women will have hot flashes in the next ten years. Talk about global warming! When millions of women are going through menopause at the same time, it's a sociological hot flash! We have to look at the effects of such an unprecedented occurrence.

When did you start yoga?

I took my first class in January 1990. I'm not one of these people who began in their twenties. I was forty-six. I started doing yoga because I had scoliosis and was experiencing some very heavy-duty back problems. Scoliosis was also a gift—without that problem I might not have discovered yoga.

I never made a conscious decision to be a yoga teacher. It was not something I planned. Everything just unfolded. Allowing things to unfold has put me where I am in my life now. It's a magical process. I don't know what's supposed to happen next. I feel like Spirit just guides me and presents opportunities.

Sometimes I say to Spirit, "Are you crazy? You want me to do what?" And then I find my courage. I step into the unknown, do it anyway and then magic happens.

God's plan is much better than any plan I could have made up. My sense is that I need to be obedient and show up 100 percent, and that's what got me to where I am. My whole life has been like this, as long as I follow my inner guidance.

How did you come to produce your video Embracing Menopause: A Path to Peace and Power?

The menopause video happened because I was going through menopause myself. I was impressed with what yoga did for me. I feel much more focused and relaxed inside because of my yoga practice. I believe that yoga was the number one reason I sailed through menopause. Through yoga, I can feel changes in my body—subtle changes that are not quantifiable.

How does your view differ from the standard medical model of menopause?

The medical paradigm of menopause has been basically an image of fear. It scares women into taking HRT (hormone replacement therapy) and thinking that if they don't they'll become dried-up, incontinent old prunes with brittle bones. Menopause is treated as a disease to be cured. But so little is known about menopause medically. The traditional medical model infuriates me! It is such a male-dominated, disempowering approach to woman's health. I really feel we have all the wisdom within us to handle our bodies and trust our inner knowing.

The current model is based upon men's historical fear of powerful women. They don't know what to do with us. The archetypal image of an intuitive, powerful, centered, Wise Woman does not exist in our culture anymore.

When you realized all this, what did you do?

I got on my bandwagon and began writing books and articles, as well as producing videos for baby boomers and for women going through menopause. I felt that if menopausal women did yoga, most of their issues could be mitigated.

Collectively, we have an opportunity to reinstate the Wise Woman in our culture. That's really the message in my classes and workshops for women going through menopause and in my menopause video—to encourage woman to take their power back, to listen to themselves and to trust their intuition. And especially to know they're not alone. They have many sisters going through the same change!

I really see yoga as a path to finding that power within, that place of knowing deep within our hearts. Unless you're in touch with your body from the inside out, you can't come from that deeper place within yourself. I see yoga as a path to connect to that power.

Susan Winter Ward is an internationally recognized yoga instructor. She received her yoga teacher's certification with Ganga White and Tracey Rich and has studied with John Friend and other leading yoga teachers in the United States. Susan leads her unique yoga workshops at retreats and conferences worldwide.

5 Yoga Builds Healthy Bones

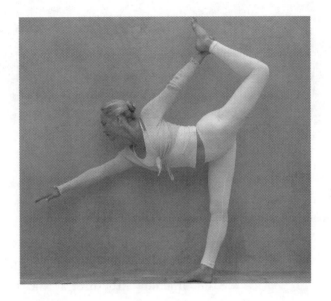

*O*steoporosis is really our magical body's
intelligent response to long-term
imbalances and stressors.

—Susan Brown, Ph.D., *Better Bones, Better Body*

*R*egular exercise is itself a powerful medicine
that helps mitigate virtually all the negative changes
women experience at midlife and beyond.

—Carol Krucoff, *Healing Moves: How to Cure,
Relieve and Prevent Common Ailments with Exercise*

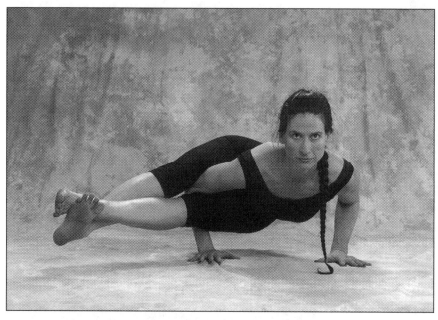

Ana Forrest in **Astavakrasana.**

The skeleton is our support system and provides the fundamental structure of the human body. Our bones enable us to stand upright and allow us to move when the muscles attached to them are contracted. Bones also protect our vital organs. The dense bones of the skull enclose the brain; the slender ribs protect the heart and lungs at the same time as they allow the chest to expand and contract.

The condition of our bones during the menopausal years reflects the converging forces of many health factors. These include our health at birth—a combination of genetics, our mother's health and her nutritional status. Equally important is our own nutritional intake and level of exercise over the years. Lifestyle factors, stress, medications, secondhand smoke, air pollution and lack of exposure to natural light are among the many

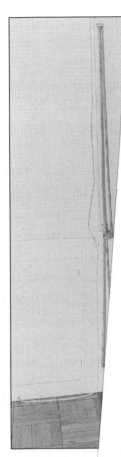
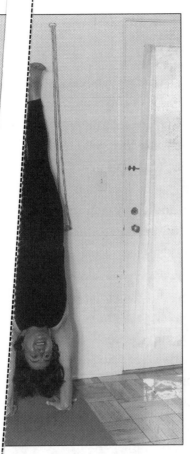

Handstands stren_____ the bones of the upper body.

environmental fac____ that affect our bone health as well.

Lifelong bone ____h is a human birthright. By working with nature, ____an maintain and even rebuild our
skeletal system. ____enturies, people who lived in harmony with natu____d who had an adequate supply of
traditional nativ____ds were not subject to osteoporosis
and other disea____ f modern civilization. When those
same people ad____ modern, fragmented eating habits,
they became s____t to modern-day degenerative diseases within a relatively short time.

Exercise literally can save your life; without it, your body deteriorates. There is no question that if you are inactive your bones will decalcify, leading to osteoporosis, the potentially fatal disease that is so prevalent among older women. Taking time out of your day to attend an exercise class, to take a walk, is not frivolous—it's essential.

—Linda Ojeda,
Menopause Without Medicine

Your Skeleton: The Body's Calcium Bank Account

Our amazing human bodies have numerous back-up systems working day and night toward keeping a relatively stable internal environment, or what is known as homeostasis.

This ability to maintain a stable internal environment, even under less than desirable conditions, allows the body to keep functioning for as long as it does. In the case of our bones, the process of homeostasis regulates the body's use of calcium.

The teeth and skeleton are particularly good storehouses for calcium. The body needs a great deal of calcium, around the clock, to maintain vital functions. Calcium is needed not just for strong bones and teeth, but also for clotting the blood, transmitting nerve impulses, ensuring muscle movement and growth, regulating the heart's rhythm and stabilizing the nervous system.

Ninety-nine percent of the body's calcium is stored in the skeleton and teeth. The remaining one percent must take care of all of calcium's other vital functions in the soft tissues of the body. If necessary, in order to meet this urgent demand, calcium is pulled from our bones. If our diet is deficient in replenishing the calcium that is used, our bones can lose up to one-third of their calcium without immediate detriment to our system.

Over time, however, this loss causes the bones to become soft and porous and may cause osteoporosis (loss of bone mass), osteopenia (low bone mass) and related degenerative disorders. These include back and disc problems, bone fractures and loss of bone surrounding the teeth (pyorrhea). From this perspective, as Susan Brown points out, osteoporosis is really the body's intelligent action in response to long-term imbalances and stresses.

Bone Density and Osteoporosis

Exploring the breakdown of the skeletal system from a broader perspective demonstrates that the underlying causes of osteoporosis go much deeper than the superficial, simplistic views promoted by pharmaceutical companies. Researchers now recognize that numerous bone-depleting factors—beyond a natural decline in estrogen at menopause and lower calcium intakes—affect bone resilience and bone health.

In fact, although osteoporosis is commonly defined as a condition of thin and fragile bones, we now know that osteoporosis and osteoporotic fractures involve more than just thin bone. And having dense bones does not guarantee freedom from fractures. Interestingly, roughly half of those with bone density low enough to qualify as having osteoporosis never experience an osteoporotic fracture. Conversely, a significant number of people with medium and even high bone density experience unexpected fractures. While mineral content and bone density are important, the ability of bone to heal and repair itself is probably of equal importance in preventing osteoporotic fractures.

Researchers have measured the bone density of people with broken bones. Twenty-five percent had osteoporosis, twenty-five percent had high bone density and fifty percent had normal bone density. People with

Generally we think of the ovaries and their hormones, estrogen and progesterone, as the most important endocrine factors influencing bone health. In truth, bone health depends on proper functioning of all the hormone-producing endocrine glands. Over- or under-functioning of the thyroid, parathyroid, adrenals, liver and kidneys can all adversely affect bone.
—Susan E. Brown, Ph.D.
Better Bones, Better Body

high bone density broke their hips as frequently as those with osteoporosis did.

Bone density readings do one thing and one thing only: read bone density. They don't measure bone strength or quality, and these also are factors that determine if bone is more likely to fracture. Bone density is measured as "mineral content per measured area unit"—or the amount of bony material in a specific space. But as Susan Love, M.D., points out in *Dr. Susan Love's Hormone Book,* "We don't in reality know what 'normal' bone density should be."

Low bone density is not necessarily a sign of brittle bone density. If bone *quality* is good, you can actually lose 25 percent or more of your bone mass and still resist fractures. In fact, it's normal to lose a bit of bone density as you get older, but that doesn't mean your bones must get brittle.

According to Dr. Christiane Northrup, women who have small bones may have low bone density because their bones have never *been* very dense—*not* because they have true osteoporosis. Consider this: a bird's bone is less dense than that of an elephant, but it is still strong enough for a bird.

Building Healthy Bones Without Drugs

While conventional medicine and the pharmaceutical industry encourage the use of various drugs for postmenopausal bone protection, numerous researchers and organizations such as the Osteoporosis Education Project (see Resources section) have concluded that, for the average woman, the risks of taking such drugs outweigh the benefits.

Both the density of bone and the ability of bone to regenerate and heal itself depend on a wide range of nutrients found only in whole, organically grown foods and in living a healthy lifestyle. In her excellent book, *Better Bones, Better Body,* author Susan E. Brown asks us to rethink the true nature and causes of osteoporosis and learn how to develop a natural life-supporting program for building and maintaining bone health.

Before taking any drug for osteoporosis, eliminate all risk factors for unhealthy, brittle bones. Keep in mind that *anything* that inhibits the body's ability to absorb calcium contributes to the likelihood of osteoporosis. Sugar is by far the main dietary culprit. Researchers have found that ingesting sugar increases the rate at which we excrete calcium. Unfortunately, taking supplemental calcium to combat this depletion, if it is not in the proper ratio to other minerals, can cause numerous other health problems, including kidney stones, bone spurs, arthritis and hardening of the arteries.

Many other substances in the modern diet affect the body's ability to absorb calcium. Ingestion of large quantities of caffeine leads to loss of calcium and other nutrients through the urine, and consumption of phosphoric acid in soft drinks causes calcium to be pulled from bones. Alcohol, smoking, aluminum from cookware and other sources, excess sodium from salt and many common medications including cold medications, anti-inflamatory drugs and steroids also interfere with calcium availability.

Make sure you receive enough vitamin D. Increasing your exposure to natural sunlight will ensure you obtain adequate doses of this essential bone-building vitamin. The vitamin D produced under your skin in sunny

The safest way to stop bone loss and maintain adequate calcium in the body is to keep the minerals in balance through proper nutrition and exercise. I have seen postmenopausal women go from secreting calcium twenty-four hours a day to normal levels within a few weeks of following healthy lifestyle guidelines. Lead a lifestyle that promotes proper mineral balance and the body will heal itself.

—Nancy Appleton, Ph.D.,
Lick the Sugar Habit

weather is stored by your body for use during the winter.

Practice weight-bearing exercise. Any kind of weight-bearing exercise sets up an electrical mini-current in your skeleton that draws strengthening minerals right into the bone matrix. In particular, increase weight-bearing standing poses and upper-body, weight-bearing poses according to your ability to practice safely. Do other healthy outdoor weight-bearing activities such as walking and playing tennis. These activities also help build bone.

The Osteoporosis "Epidemic"

Christiane Northrup, M.D., Susun Weed, Farida Sharan, Susan Love, M.D., and other health experts who have worked with menopausal women for many years, remind us that osteoporosis may not be quite the epidemic drug companies would have us believe. We all have seen the full-page ads in the media advising us to take Fosamax and, until recently, Premarin and other drugs to help build bones. These print ads are reinforced by television ads. Advertisers and many doctors tell women that they have osteoporosis when their bone density tests come back "low," and then frighten women into taking drugs that have numerous side effects, including esophageal irritation and erosion. Women on estrogen replacement therapy (ERT) to prevent osteoporosis increase their risk of breast cancer and heart attack. The health of our skeletal system is intimately involved with all the other systems of the body. A far wiser approach to good bone health is to focus on the whole body's health.

Why Yoga Is a Superior Form of Weight-Bearing Exercise

The 206 bones in the human body are living, breathing, changing tissue that require a steady supply of blood and nutrients and a flow of energy or *prana*. Yoga postures, besides providing a superior form of weight-bearing exercise that stimulates bones to retain calcium, also help stimulate and distribute the flow of synovial fluid, which lubricates the joints between the bones. Weight lifting and other forms of exercise, while strengthening bones, may cause further imbalance in the muscular system. Conversely, yoga postures balance the muscular system while bones are strengthened. When the muscular system is balanced, the skeletal system is brought back into alignment, reducing the risk of wear-and-tear conditions such as osteoarthritis.

Yoga's Weight-Bearing Benefits

- Yoga's weight-bearing poses take the body through its full range of movement.
- While other weight-bearing exercises tighten the body, yoga "lubricates" the joints by giving them an internal massage.
- Yoga builds bone strength evenly in both the upper and lower body.
- Yoga postures have a beneficial effect on the endocrine glands, which contribute to the formation of strong, healthy bones.
- Yoga has a positive effect on the adrenal glands—reducing stress levels and inhibiting excess calcium secretion.
- Yoga improves balance and coordination, helping to prevent falls.
- Yoga prevents and can even reverse the most visible and obvious symptom of osteoporosis and aging: the shortening and rounding of the spine.

Yoga is one of the few exercise systems in which weight is borne through the entire body. In weight-bearing standing poses, inverted poses, active backbends and various arm balances, weight is systematically applied to the bones in the hands, arms, upper body, neck and head, as well as the feet and legs. Inverted weight-bearing yoga poses such as Handstand, Right Angle Handstand, Elbow Balance, Headstand and Downward-Facing Dog—where the bones in the arms, wrists and hands are strengthened by supporting the weight of one's body—all work to prevent osteoporosis and other problems related to a weak skeletal structure.

These poses help strengthen the arms, upper body and upper spine. Yoga's upper-body weight-bearing poses help prevent hairline fractures in the vertebrae that cause the upper-back curvature common to older people in our culture. Because yoga postures are learned gradually, the weight applied to the bones increases safely and incrementally, as the student becomes stronger and can hold postures for longer periods.

Jan Madden, a yoga teacher who specializes in working with postmenopausal women, is also the author of *Yoga Builds Bones: Easy Gentle Stretches that Prevent Osteoporosis*. She is one of many yoga teachers who makes a strong case for weight-bearing yoga postures as the best hope of minimizing the effects of osteoporosis or preventing it altogether. In her book, Madden describes how she discovered the connection between yoga and bone strength when her mother was diagnosed with osteoporosis a decade ago. Her observation confirms my own experience working with midlife and older women for over thirty years. Madden says:

Yoga creates a balanced harmony between the ovaries, adrenals, parathyroid, pituitary and pineal gland, ensuring that the body receives a steady supply of the right hormones for maintaining bone strength and maximum health and well-being. The regular practice of weight-bearing hatha yoga postures offers women everywhere a safe, scientifically proven way to build bone strength.

Madden's book presents observational evidence from yoga teachers throughout the world to support the hypothesis that the regular practice of weight-bearing yoga prevents osteoporosis. I'm confident that in the near future the scientific community will pay attention to the evidence of yoga practitioners and begin to conduct controlled studies to prove that yoga can help prevent osteoporosis.

Yoga and the Spine

In our culture, where people spend many hours of each day engaged in activities that tend to pull the upper body forward, a rounded back, forward head and collapsed chest are so prevalent that we almost consider it normal. By the time women reach menopause, poor posture habits are often deeply ingrained, and the spine has begun to degenerate—resulting in loss of height and back and neck problems.

When the back becomes rounded, it compresses the chest and causes shallow breathing, which limits the amount of oxygen the body's cells receive. This collapsed posture contributes to cardiovascular and other health problems. Yoga counteracts and reverses all these

This is what osteoporosis means. Your inner chemical changes are occurring during menopause in such a manner that your body is becoming stiff; the spine forms a lump and it becomes crooked. The bones show the decay. So with the decaying process you have to see how you have to give fresh supply of blood to the area. You have to find out where the decaying process is occurring, where the skeletal bones are losing strength. The body becomes heavy and the spine can't bear it.

—B.K.S. Iyengar

changes, and prevents or corrects the most visible sign of osteoporosis—shortening and rounding of the spine.

Poor posture and the degeneration of the spinal column affect the health of every system of the body. Not only do a rounded spine and collapsed chest restrict breathing, they also interfere with the vital flow of blood and nerve impulses to internal organs. In this way, poor posture interferes with digestion and elimination.

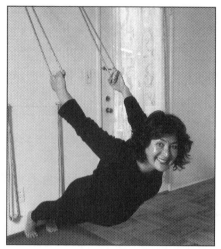

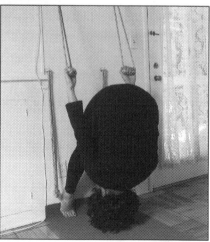

Wall ropes are the antidote to osteoporosis.

Yoga and Preventing Height Loss

According to Dr. Christiane Northrup in *Women's Bodies, Women's Wisdom,* decreased height is not always the result of bone loss. Years of poor posture, lack of stretching or feeling weighed down by life's burdens can also make a woman shorter than she once was. Some height loss results from the shrinking of spaces between vertebral discs, even when bone density is good. Dr. Northrup observed the least height loss in her patients who regularly practiced yoga. I believe this is because yoga helps keep the space between the vertebrae open, plump and supple. Many of my older students report that after practicing yoga for a while, they regain their youthful height. Similarly, when students who have experienced some height loss stand very tall and strong, the height loss is not noticeable.

Stress also contributes to osteoporosis. When we are under stress, our blood becomes slightly more acidic, which, over time, removes calcium from the bones. When we are more relaxed, our blood becomes more alkaline and doesn't loose as much calcium. The stress-reducing benefits of yoga can also help prevent osteoporosis.

Choosing a Safe Yoga Class

Women who begin yoga during menopause are advised to seek out a class appropriate to their level—one that emphasizes good body alignment and has available props to help ensure the integrity of the spine.

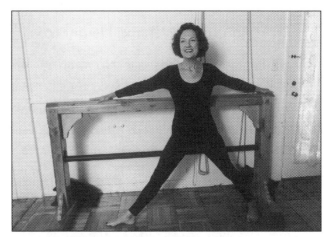

Triangle Pose (**Trikonasana**) *practiced with a bar ("horse") or other support helps create healthy body alignment.*

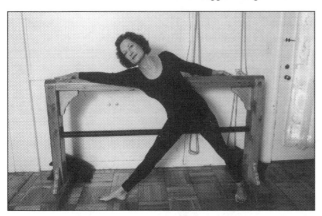

The Triangle Pose is key for preventing osteoporosis.

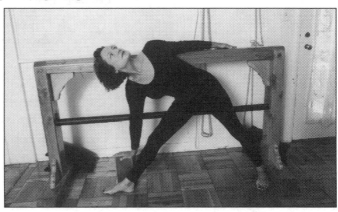

The Triangle Pose lengthens your spine and strengthens your bones.

Safe Yoga for Osteoporosis

The whole subject of osteoporosis is of increasing concern to teachers working with large numbers of students who have been told they have osteopenia or osteoporosis. Many of my women students come to yoga with concerns about the results of their bone density tests. If you are a student or teacher concerned about what yoga poses you can safely practice (or teach), I highly recommend the book, *Back Care Basics: A Doctor's Gentle Yoga Program for Back and Neck Pain Relief,* by Mary Pullig Schatz, M.D. It provides excellent guidelines on yoga for osteoporosis.

If a woman at midlife or older is new to yoga, I generally have her start with standing poses practiced with her back against a wall or windowsill or supported by a yoga prop, known as a horse or trestle, which looks similar to a gymnastic bar, to help assure good alignment.

I teach students of all ages how to move with maximum awareness, as well as how to move from their "hip hinge" with the upper body in one unit. As other teachers who are concerned about osteoporosis have pointed out, to "hinge at the hips" is the general rule. Unfortunately, stiff beginning students have a difficult time actually doing this. If the hamstring muscles at the back of the thighs are tight, it is difficult to bend forward without rounding, and consequently compressing, the back—especially in the thoracic spine, which is the area most at risk for fracture. Props are invaluable for teaching students how to lengthen the spine and create space between the discs.

Other Cautions:

- **Avoid high-impact exercise and sudden jerking, rapid movements.** High-impact exercise is hard on joints and not recommended for women who already have osteoporosis, balance problems or knee, ankle or back problems. High-impact exercise that involves bouncing while stretching, or rapid stretching with poor body alignment, may cause crush fractures of weakened vertebrae and exacerbate existing problems due to osteoporosis and poor posture.

- **Avoid activities that reinforce a rounded back (kyphosis) and/or hunched over, collapsed positions that exacerbate poor posture.** All activities where the upper body is hunched over can intensify the forces that result in vertebral crush fractures. This includes hunching over while attempting to touch your toes in a standing or seated forward bend. It is especially important for menopausal women at risk for osteoporotic fractures to practice yoga's seated poses with adequate props.

- **Avoid hyperextension of the neck.** Do not tilt the head way back. This action can potentially compress the vertebral arteries and interrupt blood flow to the brain, possibly causing fainting or even a stroke. When lying down, place adequate support under your head to keep your forehead level or slightly higher than your chin. A forward-head position and rounded upper back usually precede the vertebral wedge fractures that result in dowager's hump.

- **Avoid poses that bear weight directly on the neck.** Weak, porous vertebrae are vulnerable to injury. Women at high risk for osteoporosis should learn weight-bearing inverted poses such as

Headstand and Shoulderstand under the guidance of an experienced instructor. If you are new to yoga and have osteoporosis, Headstand and Shoulderstand are not recommended. However, Handstands, Right Angle Handstands, Dog Poses, and poses that build upper body strength without bearing weight on the vulnerable neck vertebrae can be safely learned under the guidance of an instructor.

Back Pain and Osteoporosis

Vertebral compression fractures occur most commonly in women within twenty years after menopause. Pain in the spine can be the result of muscle spasms associated with microscopic fractures of the collapsing vertebrae. Pain can be sudden and severe, or chronic and constant. With repeated tiny fractures, the vertebrae form wedges—narrow in front, wider in back—resulting in upper-back roundness. This increase in the thoracic curve is known as kyphosis or dowager's hump and includes loss of height.

The Power of Back-Strengthening Exercises

Back-strengthening exercises may help prevent fractures in women at risk for osteoporosis. A recent study published in the journal *Bone* involved fifty postmenopausal women who were not on hormone replacement therapy and did not take calcium. Half of them did back exercises for two years. After ten years, there were a third fewer vertebral fractures in the group that exercised, even though bone mineral density was comparable in both groups.

The spine gets shortened and compressed. It is not that a person grows shorter overnight. The spine shortens, the groins become stiff, the joints make noise.

—B.K.S. Iyengar

A Word on Stiffness and Starting Yoga Later in Life

People who have not exercised for many years and whose diets are heavy on sugar, caffeine, meat and processed foods commonly experience weight gain and swelling of the joints later in life. A type of stiffness may come into the body that is due not only to lack of movement but also to toxicity. Often these people find it difficult to practice yoga, but they are among those who need it the most.

In these cases, the yoga props are especially useful. Without props, people with little energy and many problems often lose heart. Props encourage the body to open and lengthen gradually. With the help of a wall, people of all ages and conditions can begin practicing the standing poses and simple inversions. Lying back on bolsters and blankets, almost everyone can practice gentle backbends. Forward bends can be practiced sitting on a prop that adds height, or with the support of a chair. Supported Lying Down Bound Angle Pose to open the groin and hips and restore energy is highly recommended.

It is important for women who feel very stiff and rigid to realize that this need not be a permanent condition. If you practice yoga faithfully, the stiffness will leave. With yoga and nutritional support, the body can be cleansed, renewed and rejuvenated. However, without healthy movement, pain and stiffness—especially if masked by medication—can settle deeper into your body, leading to arthritis, osteoporosis and other health problems.

Key Poses for Strong Bones—Preventing Osteoporosis

See chapter 8, "Yoga and the Wisdom of Menopause Practice Guide," for instructions.

Note on time: **Weight-bearing, active poses are held long enough so you strengthen but not so long that you feel strain or fatigue.** Standing poses for new students are held about half a minute each side and can be repeated several times. Experienced practitioners can hold longer. I enjoy holding Handstands for 2 minutes but for beginners 10 seconds is exhilarating.

Pose	Suggested Time
Downward- and Upward-Facing Dog Pose	1 minute
All Standing Poses	See note above
Full Arm Balance (safer than Headstand for new students—no weight bearing on neck)	See note above
Elbow Balance	according to ability
Upward-Facing Dog with Wall Ropes and Forward Bends with Wall Ropes	according to ability
Weight-Bearing Backbends	according to ability
Advanced Weight-Bearing Balance Poses	according to ability
All Restorative Poses to reduce stress	5 to 10 minutes

Gaye Abbott, age 54

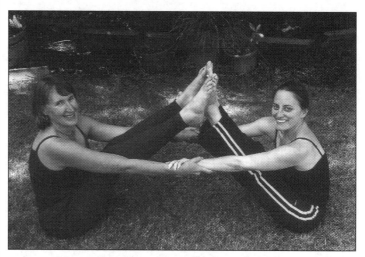

Gaye Abbott and Leza Lowitz, Partner Stretch, Boat Pose.

Deep Discoveries About Healing from Osteoporosis

At age forty-nine I was given two diagnoses—osteoporosis and a severe case of "leaky gut" syndrome. As a health care professional and yoga adept, I was stunned. The contributing factors were clear: developmentally compromised bones from an intrauterine environment of nicotine and alcohol (a common occurrence among baby boomers); secondhand smoke during childhood; huge amounts of antibiotics for teenage acne (there go the good guys in the digestive system); a total hysterectomy for endometriosis at age thirty-two; and an emotional roller coaster of a life, centered on helping others and being the one to "hold it all together" (nurse, massage therapist, single parent of three boys).

Many questions arose for me in the process of healing. How does one become resilient and sustain a high level of health, all the way down to the bones? What relationship did I have with my bones (alive or dead)? Why had my digestive system been invaded and become unable to absorb? Why was it leaking out the nutrients that I needed for a strong foundation? What engrained patterns of living did I need to examine? Where was I lacking support? What was my body telling me?

I discovered that it wasn't so important to find answers for these questions. Rather, the process of raising them provided a stimulus to *pay attention,* which invariably led to more exploration. This was meditation in action! The process was alive, and I became alive within it. I dove beneath the fear-based medical system and realized that my body's wisdom had brought me an opportunity to examine the whole of my life and expand my playing field.

The deeper discoveries took time and are continuing to emerge. They unfold within my yoga practice and teaching, as well as in my relationships, professional choices, behavior patterns and inner dialogue. I recognized that I had been living with the assumption that life takes more than it gives—a process of total depletion! My yoga practice became a means to disassemble the blueprint of illusion that I had constructed for my life.

I learned that living wasn't about *doing* all the "right things," such as diet, nutritional supplements, herbal hormonal creams and weight-bearing exercise. Instead, it was about *paying attention* and *being present* in all the moments of my life—yoga practice on and off the mat! It meant saying yes! from a place of authentic curiosity—saying yes! to creating, playing, trying new things, taking risks, making mistakes, accepting the support of other people, thriving within my life as reflected in the aliveness in the very marrow of my bones.

Part of what emerged over the past two years came in the form of a creative endeavor with women's yoga retreats. Most of the women attending are in their forties and fifties, but I am also blessed with some in their sixties and seventies. In this setting, teaching and practicing yoga have taken on an entirely new dimension, one in which each moment holds the opportunity for creation and stepping out of the "boxes" that bind us. We practice, breathe, meditate, dance, sing, write, play and reveal ourselves to one another. The walls come "tumbling down," and a collective sigh of relief is heard all over.

At age fifty-four you will find me saying, "I don't know" to a student or colleague; throwing myself into Half Moon Pose while waiting in those long bathroom lines; singing a few lines from a love song with the post office clerk while buying stamps; smiling at strangers and handing them See's chocolates—just because; engaging with a ninety-four-year-old man—encountered while walking around a local lake—and asking him with curiosity what he thinks of death; breaking into a funky dance step in the midst of my "power walk" on a busy hiking trail; requesting my yoga students (in my best southern belle voice) to share what they need in class by taking on another persona; remaining quiet when all I want to do is talk, and talking when all I want to do is melt into my surroundings; welcoming disorientation; being completely honest; meditating daily—any place, any position; falling in love all the time, all over the place—and letting people know; considering a six-month sabbatical in Italy for my fifty-fifth year; coming to my senses—taste! . . . smell! . . . touch! . . . listen! . . . breathe!

Now picture a row of tract homes that you can see from the freeway. Most of them blend together, one into the next, in their neutral colors. The bright yellow one in the middle used to make you smile, but now it has faded and doesn't stand out quite so much. But wait, you spy a newcomer! A brilliant, electric blue house, solidly built, amidst the sea of compliance and mediocrity. The electric blue house is me!

Gaye Abbott is a teacher of yoga and a leader of women's retreats. She is dedicated to the practice of yoga as a vehicle to move into the larger field of life without illusion. Blending curiosity and play, she steps off into the void and sometimes falls on her face. Gaye says, "Life is not lived in isolation; it's a group thing, a hoedown! Come play with me!"

Elizabeth Memel, age 61

Yoga Strengthened My Bones After Radiation for Breast Cancer

My passion is my work with families as an infant developmental specialist. I facilitate parenting classes both at my private studio in Ojai and at the Iyengar Yoga Institute of Los Angeles. The gift of hatha yoga has enabled me to stay physically and energetically fit so I can move easily up and down and along the floor in my work. Through yoga and my career path, I am rejuvenated—made to feel, appear and become young again.

I have been concerned about osteoporosis since my mother suffered a broken hip in an "osteoporosis fall" from which she never really recovered. I went for my first bone density test at age fifty, wanting to get a baseline measurement so I could monitor my health more effectively by keeping informed. I discovered there was already a significant gap between the medical standard and the condition of my body.

During this time, I had been studying Iyengar yoga for about seven years. I received tremendous benefits from these classes—physically, spiritually and psychologically. But after the results of the bone density test, I decided to redouble my efforts to see how much I could improve in this area. I began taking four classes a week instead of two, including a weeklong Iyengar yoga intensive with Manouso Manos in Hawaii. (What a memorable, rejuvenating experience that was, with my twenty-three-year-old daughter alongside me!)

In 1996, at age fifty-five, after five years along this path, my second bone density test was the proof of my effort. The numbers showed that the discrepancy between my body and the standard, which was for a thirty-year-old body, had been cut in half compared to what it was five years before. All those weight-bearing standing and inverted poses had paid off in a very big way!

This is very important for women concerned about having healthy bones: Doubling my yoga practice halved the discrepancy of my bone density. Another five years later, in 2000, at age fifty-nine, a third test showed I was not losing any ground. This was amazing considering I had battled breast cancer in the meantime.

The diagnosis of breast cancer placed me with a growing, looming sector of women drawn into an abyss of struggle and fear. I had to find my way through weeks of hunting for answers so I could make an informed choice. With guidance and support from loving family and caring doctors, I decided my choices were a lumpectomy—which was, frankly, not that hard—and then, in sheer resignation, radiation a few weeks postsurgery.

A few days after the surgery I met with Bonnie Anthony, a senior Iyengar yoga teacher and a breast cancer survivor, who generously showed me so much that I could do to benefit my healing. She shared the guidance she had personally received from B.K.S. Iyengar. But even with her skilled, kind inspiration, I felt myself faltering perilously because I had grave doubts about going on with the conventional medical approach. I had followed alternative healing practices for over twenty years, so my constant search for answers, often until 2:00 A.M. on the Internet, was inevitable.

Three weeks passed and my dreaded appointment for the radiation prep was coming. The day before, I hoped to return to a yoga class with my wonderful teacher in Los Angeles, Leslie Peters. I was so driven to be there that I had to run out of the house with a wet head of hair in order to get there on time. The class began with some rather simple stretches, which I gladly modified to protect myself, mostly reveling in the fact that I had gotten myself there at all. After about twenty minutes, it was time for the rest of the class to dig deeper, and I had to lie low on the fringe. It seemed totally appropriate, so I accepted my limited allowance.

My caring teacher was most solicitous, but then turned to the others to conduct their rigorous practice in her own joyous, uplifting style. As I listened to her voice, I began to feel myself react to the separation. I became upset by the fact that I was indeed deprived of participating in this very important piece of my former life—and it was the cancer that had robbed me. I started to weep silently. I became so angry at my state that I found my mind grasping at the prospect of the radiation with a vengeance. I knew right then that I would embrace most wholeheartedly whatever it would take to end this cancer siege! I was finally ready and able to choose the treatment that would assure my return to good health.

Last year, the bone density test was performed again, and the results were close to normal. I'm determined to get back on track by increasing my weekly hours of practice.

Elizabeth Memel, M.A., is committed to Iyengar yoga and takes classes at the B.K.S. Iyengar Yoga Institute of Los Angeles as well as with Suza Francina in Ojai. Yoga helps her to work with infants and toddlers in a demonstration program called RIE (Resources for Infant Educarers). One of the goals of this program is authentic development of motor skills from birth, thus fostering healthy musculoskeletal function for life.

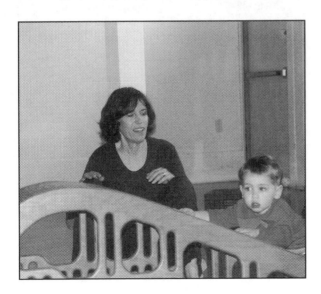

6 Yoga for Coping with Cancer

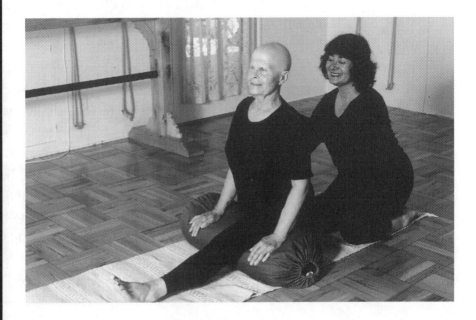

We can "do everything right" and still get sick. With yoga, we inwardly search for true healing of body, mind and spirit, not just a "cure" for our physical body. We learn to consciously heal ourselves and live. None of us knows how long that precious time will last. We train ourselves to be fully aware and conscious when we meet life's challenges.

—NISCHALA JOY DEVI, *THE HEALING PATH OF YOGA*

A NOTE TO READERS: *Photos of Malchia Olshan appear throughout this chapter. Since the photos were taken, her hair is growing back and all signs indicate she is on the road to recovery.*

I see yoga as a resource. You can use it for stress management, as a powerful ally in a storm, or a vehicle for profound self-acceptance, transformation, and love.

—Esther Myers, yoga teacher, breast cancer survivor, *Yoga Journal*, October 2001; producer of the video *Gentle Yoga for Breast Cancer Survivors*

Yoga philosophy recognizes that every human being has a unique personal path to self-realization. Likewise, yoga is supportive and respectful of the fact that when we are faced with illness, each of us has to investigate for ourselves and find out what path to healing will most serve us. This is especially relevant in the case of life-threatening illness such as cancer.

Many cancer patients have found yoga very effective in increasing their capacity to manage stress. Women who practice yoga after being diagnosed with a serious illness like cancer often say, "No matter how lousy I feel, the yoga makes me feel better." There is ample anecdotal evidence that during times of illness, yoga helps reduce levels of stress and brings about a feeling of peace and well-being. A regular yoga practice can help us tap into our inner reserves and give us the equanimity that is so needed during difficult times in our life. Yoga can enhance the quality of life when coping with cancer.

The Current Status of Cancer Research and Treatment

Many doctors and other health professionals have pointed out that the real cure for most modern diseases, including cancer, is to remove carcinogenic substances from the air, water and food supply, and to do everything possible to enhance our own body's defenses. The vast majority of cancers are causally related to the high levels of chemicals released into our air, water, soil and food over the past fifty years. United States government researchers estimate that 80 percent of all cancers are environmentally linked.*

---

* *"The Yoga of Breast Health" by Joanna Colwell, www.ottercreekyoga.com. See Resources.*

Unfortunately, current cancer research tends to focus on treating cancer at the cellular level rather than preventing it. While this research has yielded various treatments for women with existing cancers, it has little to offer healthy women in the way of resources for keeping healthy and cancer-free. While mammograms, Pap smears and other tests may help detect cancer, they will not prevent it.

This chapter focuses primarily on breast cancer, but the principles expressed apply to many other forms of cancer as well. It is beyond the scope of this book to discuss all the dimensions involved in the prevention and cure of cancer. While there are many aspects of cancer beyond our control, it makes sense to do our best to prevent cancer and other illnesses by nourishing our body with food that is organically grown and boosting our immune system with yoga and other healing practices.

> Yoga encourages us to take the deep view and the wide view. True prevention will only happen when we identify the causes of cancer and remove those causes.
>
> —Joanna Colwell, "The Yoga of Breast Health"

Practicing Yoga to Reduce Breast Cancer Risk

Clinical studies over the past decade are starting to demonstrate that moderate activity, intelligently adjusted to an individual's abilities and energy level, can be of great value in healing cancer patients. The practice of yoga, therefore, can play an important role as part of a healthy lifestyle aimed at reducing the risk of breast cancer. Yoga can also enhance healing and recovery if cancer has been diagnosed.

Yoga can help reduce the risk of breast cancer by stimulating lymph flow, strengthening the endocrine and immune systems, and helping you be more in touch with your body.

Yoga can begin to create an inner environment that prepares the ground for healing. It is as if, when we clear away the mental debris through yoga and meditation, our being breathes a sigh of relief, and the residual energy alive in us is allowed to grow and flourish. We empower this most vital and elemental part of ourselves when we hold still, when we pay attention. Some would call this process spiritual. All of us, whatever our beliefs, can recognize this state of grace, this moment of freedom. Yoga teachers can show us how to cultivate this healing condition, give us the physical and mental tools, even when we are gravely ill, to access our deepest, most sustaining energy.

—Sandy Boucher, "Yoga for Cancer," *Yoga Journal,* May/June 1999

The tissues of the breasts—glands, ducts, connective tissue and fat cells—begin to grow rapidly in response to the hormonal changes that happen at puberty. Throughout a woman's life, the complex hormonal balance regulated by the endocrine system—including the ovaries and pancreas; the pineal, pituitary, thyroid, parathyroid, adrenal and thymus glands; and other scattered tissues—has an enormous impact on the development and health of the breasts.

Stress can disrupt the endocrine (glandular) system. In addition, the liver and kidneys must be healthy for proper estrogen levels to be maintained. If too much estrogen is produced, or if the body isn't using estrogen efficiently, the liver must break down the excess and send it to the kidneys to be flushed from the system. If the liver is overworked from dealing with too many toxins, the excess estrogen is reabsorbed back into the bloodstream—and the body has more of the hormone than it can use.

As we explored in chapter 2, yoga practice contributes to our health by regulating the endocrine system and thus the balance of hormones to which we're exposed. Yoga also strengthens the immune system, especially by stimulating the flow of lymphatic fluids. Yoga provides both a philosophy and practice for creating a healthy relationship between our bodies and the world around us.

The yoga practices suggested in this book support the endocrine glands in maintaining an optimal balance of hormones in the body. Inversions help keep all systems of the body healthy, including the immune system—the body's defense mechanism. A number of critical glands—the pineal, thyroid, parathyroid and thymus— are located in the head, neck and chest. Inverted poses are believed to improve circulation to these glands, which can then work better.

Our immune system also plays a major role in protecting us from breast cancer and other forms of cancer. Inverted yoga poses are considered especially beneficial for immune function. Safe, supported poses, such as Legs Up the Wall, are highly recommended. All restorative poses, which are ideal for replenishing our reserves when we are ill or depleted, are also recommended for strengthening the immune system.

Yoga for Breast Health

Yoga helps strengthen another component of our immune system: the lymphatic system. Lymph is the

> Yoga is not a magical practice to elude death. It is a tool to help us improve the quality of each moment, of each exquisite moment, and go graciously to our merging with the infinite when our time has come.
> —Nischala Joy Devi,
> *The Healing Path of Yoga*

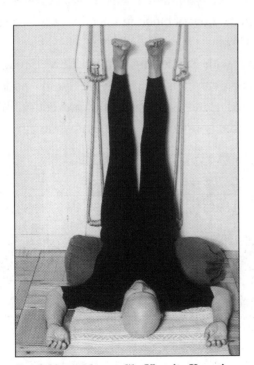

Restful inverted poses like **Viparita Karani,** *are beneficial for immune function.*

Inasmuch as the physical, mental, and spiritual practices of yoga that lead to inner transformation can help us heal at many levels, the cancer patient is advised by the most fundamental teaching of yoga that there is no single right way to do this.
—Michael Lerner,
Choices in Healing: Integrating the Best of Conventional and Complementary Approaches to Cancer

clear fluid that drains from around the body's cells into the lymphatic system, a network of thin-walled vessels found throughout every organ and tissue of your body. Lymph depends upon the muscles in the body to keep it flowing. Exercise increases the circulation of lymph fluids in the body, which helps boost our immune system.

Just like our bodies, our cells take in nutrients and excrete wastes. If lymphatic fluid doesn't flow, cells are surrounded by their own waste. Bathed in cellular debris and toxins, the body's cells cannot receive proper nutrition.

Unlike the blood, which is pumped through the body by the heart, lymph flow depends on the muscles of the body to keep it flowing. Many kinds of movement can help circulate lymphatic fluids: massage, deep breathing and even the flow of blood in a nearby vein. Yoga improves lymph flow.

Along with supporting lymph flow throughout the body, yoga can help stimulate the lymph nodes. These specialized glands, central to the prevention of disease, manufacture lymphocytes (a type of white blood cell) and

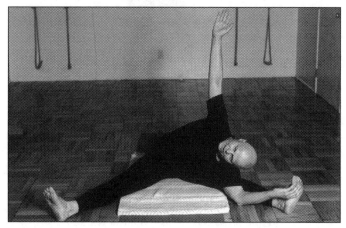

Preparation for Revolved Seated Wide Angle Pose.

filter wastes and other unwanted matter from lymph fluid. The largest clusters of lymph nodes in the body are located in the armpits, adjacent to the breasts.

Many yoga poses contract and stretch the muscles of the chest, arms and shoulders—massaging nearby lymph nodes and encouraging lymph flow through the area. Gentle Floor Twists stretch the armpits and can easily be modified, if necessary, by placing folded blankets under the legs or arms. Supported backbends over a bolster can also be very effective at gently stretching and stimulating this area.

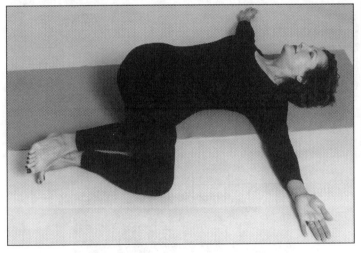

Gentle Floor Twist.

Yoga Poses for Women in Breast Cancer Treatment

Conventional treatments currently available to women with breast cancer have uncomfortable side effects. Chest surgery causes stiffness and soreness in many areas, including the upper back. If you begin yoga after surgery, search for a teacher who understands your situation, and preferably begin with private sessions or take a specialized class or workshop. Be sure to inform the teacher of your physical condition before taking a group class.

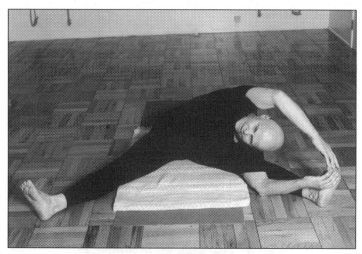

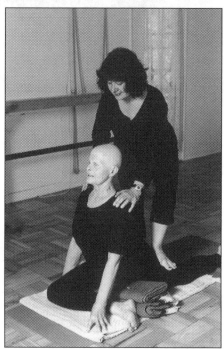

Stress and Cancer

Over the past four decades, experimental studies have demonstrated that stress influences the immune system and contributes to the development and progress of immune-based diseases such as cancer and AIDS. A landmark 1989 study by Stanford psychiatrist David Spiegel, M.D., found that women with metastatic breast cancer who participated in a support group lived longer than those who did not. The group support was seen to protect against or lessen stress. Likewise, yoga, breathing exercises and meditation can reduce stress and promote healing.

A number of physician-directed programs, such as Dean Ornish's Prostate Cancer Lifestyle Trial and the Breast Cancer Personal Support and Lifestyle Integration Program in San Francisco, train patients in yoga postures, breathing and meditation techniques.

Cancer-help retreats offer intensive contact and support. In addition, some individual yoga instructors are adapting their teachings for patients limited by illness or disability. In these settings, yoga teachers work individually with their cancer patient students. They have learned to be extremely sensitive to special needs, to maintain strong, open communication with the patient and to creatively adapt postures and other yogic elements. Practicing the postures enhances the physical benefits of yoga to a cancer patient—including range of motion, flexibility, strength, relaxation and a sense of physical well-being. But there is an additional, more mystical, benefit of yoga.

Experienced yoga teachers recognize that managing one's cancer can be a difficult task. For someone with cancer, even with consistent support from family and friends, each day can be a struggle. Yoga can offer a healing respite from this struggle. It offers a way to step out of the cycle of pain and depletion and to transcend— even for brief moments—the often unrelenting struggle someone coping with cancer experiences. The value of this brief transcendence cannot be overestimated.

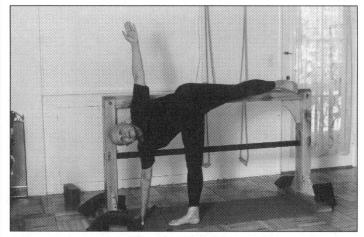

Half Moon Pose on the horse. A yoga prop called the "horse" allows standing poses to be practiced while conserving precious energy reserves.

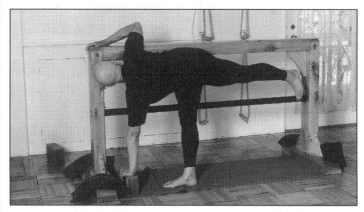

Revolved Half Moon Pose.

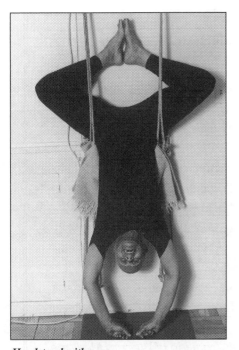

Headstand with rope.

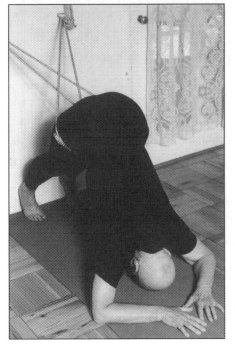

Shoulderstand with a chair.

Downward-Facing Dog Pose with rope. The entire weight of the body is taken by the rope so that there is no strain and the benefits of the pose can be obtained even during times of illness and low energy.

Good Reading and Resources

Books:

An Alternative Medicine Guide to Cancer, by Burton Goldberg

Breast Cancer? Breast Health! The Wise Woman Way, by Susun S. Weed

Choices in Healing: Integrating the Best of Conventional and Complementary Approaches to Cancer, by Michael Lerner

Dr. Susan Love's Breast Book, by Susan Love, M.D.

The Path of Practice: A Woman's Book of Ayurvedic Healing, by Bri. Maya Tiwari

The Wisdom of Menopause, by Christiane Northrup, M.D.; chapter on "Creating Breast Health"

A Matter of Health: Integration of Western Medicine in Prevention and Cure, by Dr. Krishna Raman

Internet:

www.drweilselfhealing.com, self-healing Web site of Andrew Weil, M.D.

Videos:

Gentle Yoga for Breast Cancer Survivors, with Esther Myers

Yoga and the Gentle Art of Healing: A Journey of Recovery After Breast Cancer, with Susan Rosen

(Please see the Resources section for ordering information and additional yoga and cancer resources.)

Key Poses for a Healthy Immune System

See chapter 8, "Yoga and the Wisdom of Menopause Practice Guide," for instructions.

Reminder: Do not be in a hurry. Select only the number of poses you can do without feeling rushed. **Time suggested is the minimum time.** Experienced practitioners can stay in poses longer.

Pose	Suggested Time
Supported Lying Down Bound Angle Pose	10 minutes
Downward-Facing Dog Pose Hanging in Ropes or Supported	2 minutes
Supported Shoulderstand	2 to 5 minutes
Plow Pose	2 to 5 minutes
Supported Legs Up the Wall Pose	10 minutes
All Inverted Poses	according to ability
Lying Back Over a Chair or Backbender	according to ability
Deep Relaxation Pose (Supported or with Bolster Under Legs)	5 minutes or longer

Catherine Meek, age 56

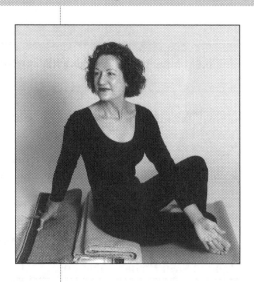

Ahhh, Yoga—It Kept Me Sane and Made Me Whole Again

I was forty-six years old when I was diagnosed with an aggressive breast cancer tumor. I was an otherwise healthy individual with no history of breast cancer in my family.

Initially, I resisted the traditional treatment of "slash, burn and poison"—until I researched the statistics. If I didn't follow this traditional course, my chances for survival were not good.

My treatment consisted of chemotherapy, radiation and five years of Tamoxifen medication. After my first chemotherapy treatment, I went into immediate menopause—a condition known in breast cancer circles as crash "chemopause." Imagine all the menopausal symptoms that are supposed to occur gradually in your body happening in one week, all at the same time!

I realized my life was in for some major changes one day as I was making a presentation to about 200 people. Out of nowhere, my make-up came streaming down my face and my lovely silk suit was completely soaked! Tough to keep one's cool in that situation. It was then that I decided I had to take control of my body. I researched everything I could find and started on a regimen of diet, herbs, visualization and yoga.

Ahhh, yoga! It kept me sane and made me whole again. I started with restorative yoga during treatment. These poses helped me work through the worst of the chemotherapy and helped relax and calm me for the next round. I wasn't strong enough to do many of the asanas, but my teacher helped me see the healing and spiritual aspects of yoga.

What really made me understand the wonders of yoga practice, however, was the impact yoga had on my bone density. Due to chemotherapy, I had lost 45 percent of the bone mass in my spine and hips. I was on medication, which did increase it. But as soon as I stopped the medication, my bone density decreased. Now, after five years of consistent yoga practice, the bone density has increased again.

Yoga has not only helped ease many of my physical symptoms, particularly through menopause, it also makes me feel strong. I like being a "warrior." I feel powerful when I do a backbend, and—oh, did I like the feeling of strength when I finally kicked up into a handstand!

Yoga has enhanced my life—physically, emotionally and spiritually. Now, at age fifty-six, ten years after I was diagnosed with breast cancer, I am grateful and blessed to have found it.

Namasté.

Catherine Meek is president of Meek and Associates and has practiced in the compensation field for over thirty years. She consults with entrepreneurial organizations and Fortune 500 companies. As a breast cancer survivor, Catherine's volunteer activities include working with the National Breast Cancer Coalition (www.stopbreastcancer.org). She is married to the world's best husband, Al Earle, and lives in Ojai, California, where she loves to practice yoga, walk, read, learn piano, and listen to rock and roll.

Maggie Mellor, age 55

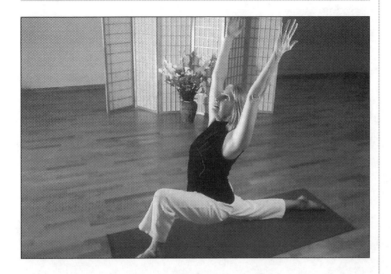

We live in tumultuous times, and all of us face uncertainty, personally and collectively. Yoga offers tools and practices to let go of old ways of being; connect with our deepest self; set intentions; and find stability in this rapidly changing world.
—Maggie Mellor, yoga teacher

My Journey Through Breast Cancer—
How Yoga Helped Me

It should never have happened to me. I am a yoga teacher, health conscious and mostly vegetarian for the last thirty years.

In my hospital gown, I stood defiantly before the famous Dr. Giulano at the John Wayne Cancer Clinic in January 1998. It was my fiftieth year. "I am 99 percent certain," I spouted, "that this is not cancer!" He paused, looked me in the eyes and responded with, "And I am 50 percent certain that it is."

This rather threw my bravado off balance, and I agreed to a biopsy. Cancer it was. My husband and I were unable to speak as we were left alone in the room to drink in the terrible news. Within a few days, the small lump and the surrounding areas were surgically removed. Thankfully, I lost only one or two lymph nodes.

Three months down the line, I had completed radiation and considered myself done with the medical model. Now what? If this had happened to me, it could happen to anyone. This stealthy thief in the night that could rob me of my life needed to be examined. I set about consulting various practitioners to resolve the matter. I now examine everything I eat, drink, do, say and think with a fine-tooth comb. So what toxicity lingers in me? What emotional pattern is eating me up from the inside?

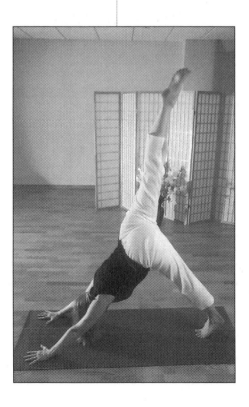
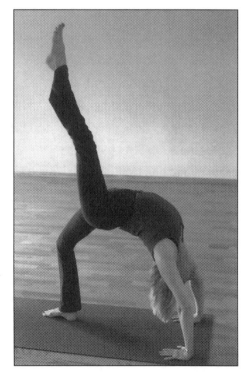

I still don't really know what caused this, but thanks to that very stabilizing and centering practice that yoga offered me throughout the ordeal, I was able to swim—at times just float—and be carried through the stormy times. I'll never forget sitting on my mat a few days after the lumpectomy—I was longing to do a spinal twist. In the hospital, lying in bed and wearing that enormous supportive bra they issue, my body had felt stiff and weak. I wanted to enliven it. I wanted to feel the life force flow through me again.

Eventually, I needed more than the physical movements. As my body healed, and my medical treatments came to an end, my mood began to drop. What now?

I have been attending yoga classes with Rod Stryker over the years, and I had completed his advanced teacher training program. I consulted Rod, and together we developed a strong daily practice of *pranayama*. Twenty minutes every day of *Pratiloma Ujjayi*. This is a variation of alternate nostril breathing that brings balance and calm. And it requires great concentration to do properly! I gradually increased the length of the exhaled breath until it was four times as long as the inhaled breath.

This is very calming and stilling to the thoughts. Silence follows—and I am able to hold that stillness in the pause at the end of the exhale. Out of this stillness I am able to experience my body as an energy field, radiant with light. I hold this image, letting the radiant light stream through me.

Maggie Mellor has thirty years of yoga experience, and has explored, through the ancient teachings, the new dimensions in human consciousness. She has studied in the Shivananda, Iyengar and Pure Yoga Schools of Yoga. Maggie was born in Holland and raised in South Africa. She has lived in Europe, Japan and Australia, and currently lives and teaches in Southern California.

7 Yoga for a Woman's Heart

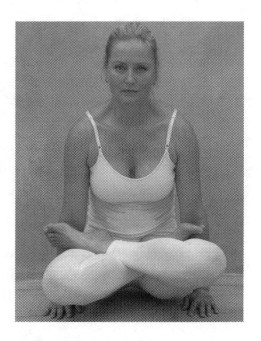

*The human heart is not sealed off from
countless processes that take place within the human
body. It is a point of culmination, a collection center
for all the malfunctions or deficiencies that exist
in the body as a whole. It is a zone of infinite
vulnerability to all the anguishes and insults and
provocations of mind, soul and body.*

—NORMAN COUSINS, *THE HEALING HEART*

145

We don't know where the soul is in the body . . . there's actually a piece of tissue in the heart that touches all four chambers. And the heart really is that entity for me—its power, strength, energy and spirit.

—Mehmet Oz, M.D., *Healing from the Heart: A Leading Surgeon Combines Eastern and Western Traditions to Create the Medicine of the Future*

A Woman's Heart:
Where Body, Mind and Spirit Converge

The heart is the organ that pumps blood to all parts of the body. It is located in the thoracic cavity, nestled between the lungs. The circulatory system—composed of arteries, veins and capillaries—carries blood to the heart and from the heart to the entire body, supplying oxygen and nutrients to the body's organs, cells, and tissues and carrying away waste products.

Often incorrectly called "a man's disease," heart disease—or more correctly, cardiovascular disease (CVD)—is the number one killer of women in the United States; roughly 45 percent of all female deaths are the result of CVD. According to the American Heart Association, CVD, particularly coronary heart disease and stroke, claims the lives of more than 500,000 women in America and other developed countries every year—more than breast cancer *plus* the next 15 causes of death combined.

Cardiovascular disease kills by means of both heart attack and stroke. Heart attacks alone kill almost 240,000 women each year, and women who suffer heart attacks are more likely to die from them than are men. Forty-four percent of women (compared with 27 percent of men) will die within one year of having a heart attack.

One of the major reasons women are less likely to recover from heart attacks than men is that until recently, treatment of cardiovascular disease in women was based on what physicians knew about men. Therefore, women were often misdiagnosed or diagnosed later than their male counterparts, which limited their treatment options.

The years around menopause are the time when a woman's risk for heart disease, hypertension (high blood pressure) and stroke increase significantly. Because the incidence of heart disease in women rises at about the same time that estrogen levels decrease, scientists have long assumed that heart disease after menopause is related to estrogen deficiency. Consequently, until very recently, doctors routinely prescribed estrogen replacement therapy (ERT) not only to relieve menopausal symptoms but for its supposed protection against heart disease.

The Women's Health Initiative Study found that hormone replacement therapy (HRT) in healthy women may actually increase the risk for heart attacks and is no longer recommended for long-term use in the prevention of heart disease. In addition, the particular combination HRT pill studied carried small but significant increased risks for conditions such as breast cancer, stroke and blood clots. (For the latest information on the myriad of questions about HRT, the numerous other brands of estrogen and progestin and the so-called designer estrogens and related HRT products on the market, see the alternative and conventional menopause Web sites listed in the Resource section.)

Differences Between Women and Men in Heart Disease

The symptoms of heart disease in women are often ignored, unrecognized or misdiagnosed, because women's symptoms can be different from men's. According to cardiologist Nieca Goldberg, M.D., chief of cardiac rehabilitation and chief of the Women's Heart

Program at Lenox Hill Hospital in New York, heart problems in women differ from those in men, beginning with the warning signs. While chest pain, tightness and pressure mark the classic signs of a heart attack in men, women need to watch for other often missed signals, such as unusual fatigue, shortness of breath, nausea or dizziness, lower chest or upper abdominal discomfort and back pain.

Women can often distinguish these early warning signs from ordinary aches and pains by noticing the circumstances in which they occur. When these symptoms are connected to heart disease, they often first appear when women exert themselves. After a time, the pain may worsen to the point where it occurs while at rest or sleeping. Experts advise women who suspect something might be wrong not to ignore these symptoms and to have them checked out before they worsen. Because of missed diagnoses and undertreatment, women under the age of 75 are twice as likely as men to die from heart disease.

Mehmet Oz, M.D., one of the nation's leading heart surgeons and author of *Healing from the Heart,* points out that women's hearts are physically different from men's. The standard model for heart attacks, in which the arteries get clogged and blood flow to the heart is cut off, is not the norm for women. The arteries that provide blood flow to the heart muscle are like rigid pipes in men, according to Dr. Oz, while women's are soft. Only 30 percent of women who suffer from heart disease have calcium build-up or plaque in their arteries, whereas for men the corresponding figure is 90 percent.

Heart attacks in women often occur when the arteries have a spasm and shrink. This spasm interrupts the flow of blood into the heart, which damages the muscle.

In *Healing from the Heart,* Dr. Oz cites cases demonstrating that emotional stress is more likely to precipitate cardiac arrest in women than physical stress, which is a far more common factor in men. Emotional stress often causes an adrenaline rush that produces an increase in blood pressure and heart rate. For women already susceptible to coronary artery disease, this can trigger a shortage of blood flow to the heart and increase the risk of death.

Women respond to stress differently than men do. Research shows that friendships between women can actually counteract the stress most of us experience in our everyday lives. A landmark UCLA study suggests that woman respond to stress with brain chemicals that cause us to make and maintain friendships with other women. Until this study was published, scientists generally believed that stress triggered a hormonal cascade that prepares the body to either stand and fight or to flee as fast as possible. Five decades of stress research—most of it on men—supported the theory that this fight-or-flight mechanism was left over from primitive times.

Now researchers suspect that women have a stress response mechanism that goes beyond just fight or flight. According to Laura Cousino Klein, Ph.D., an assistant professor of biobehavioral health at Pennsylvania State University, it seems that when the hormone oxytocin is released as part of the stress response in a woman, it buffers the fight-or-flight response and encourages her to tend children and gather with other women instead. When she actually engages in this tending or befriending, studies suggest that more oxytocin is released, which further counters stress and produces a calming effect.

My longest journey into the country of healing and self-renewal began with a single step, which was my recognition that I had survived a very serious heart attack. No longer could I delude myself that it was anything less than that. No longer could I believe, as I had always believed, that women were immune to heart disease, unless they were born with a damaged heart, [that it] was a men-only disease, as so many of my friends who had husbands with damaged hearts also believed.

—Pat Biondi Krantzler, M.A., *The Heart of a Woman: A Memoir of Healing and Reversing Heart Disease*

We all have twenty-four hours in a day. How much time during your day are you willing to dedicate to keeping yourself well? Is it time to reevaluate your priorities as if your life depended on it? It does!

—Nischala Joy Devi, *The Healing Path of Yoga: Time-Honored Wisdom and Scientifically Proven Methods That Alleviate Stress, Open Your Heart and Enrich Your Life*

Dr. Klein and others discovered that by not including women in stress research, scientists may have made a big mistake! Study after study has found that social ties reduce our risk of disease by lowering blood pressure, heart rate and cholesterol. There is no doubt that having friends adds to our health and longevity.

In both men and women, heart disease is highly individual. For example, someone with relatively little obstruction in the coronary arteries can be incapacitated by squeezing chest pains (angina), while another person with more severely obstructed arteries may not even be aware of a problem. Some people have run marathons with 85 percent of their coronary arteries blocked; others with no outward sign of arteriosclerosis have dropped dead of heart attacks. Physical causes alone explain only a portion of heart disease.

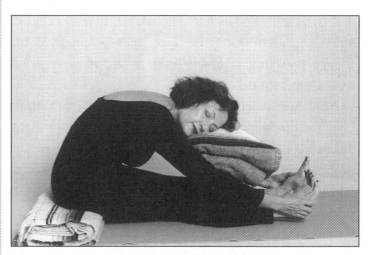

In animals, the spine is parallel to the ground and the heart is below the spine. In humans, the spinal column is perpendicular to the ground. Because of our upright position, we are more prone to strain on and diseases of the heart. In Seated Forward Bends, the spine is parallel to the ground so that the heart can rest.

Yoga for Heart Health

Yoga expert Krishna Raman, M.D., says that in *Viparita Karani,* "The blood flow collects in the pelvis and this spills over like a waterfall to the heart, flushing open the cardiac vessels."

According to Dr. Krishna Raman and other yoga experts, passive, supported backbends such as *Viparita Dandasana,* gently stretch the heart muscle and the cardiac vessels that supply the heart. This increases blood flow to the heart and helps prevent arterial blockages. Backbends also help maintain the elasticity of blood vessels and force the heart to contract—lengthening cardiac muscle and enhancing blood flow. The most important task of the cardiovascular system is to supply blood to the brain. Inverted poses help strengthen the heart, increase blood flow to the brain and may prevent the death of brain cells.

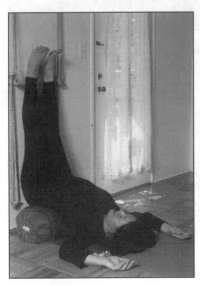

Viparita Karani.

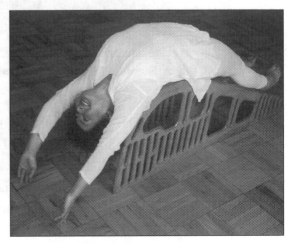

Viparita Dandasana *on the backbender.*

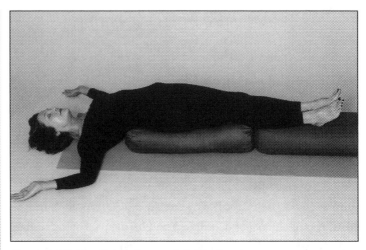

Supported Bridge Pose helps regulate blood pressure.

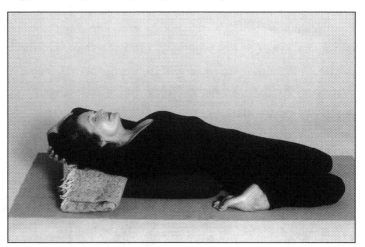

Supported Lying Down Hero Pose.

The chest opening in the restful, supported variation of the Supported Lying Down Hero Pose is particularly beneficial for the heart. Supported Lying Down Hero Pose helps prevent arterial blockages by gently massaging and strengthening the heart and increasing coronary blood flow. It stretches the abdomen, aids digestion, relieves acidity and flatulence and is one of the few poses that can be done after a heavy meal. This pose also helps relieve discomfort and swelling in the legs and feet and helps prevent varicose veins. Caution: If you have chest pains (angina) or partially blocked arteries, or are recovering from bypass surgery, practice this pose only under the guidance of a knowledgeable teacher.

Taking Your Emotions to Heart

William Harvey, the father of modern heart physiology, understood over 300 years ago that the mind and emotions affect the health of the heart. As he put it, "Every affection of the mind that is attendant with either pain or pleasure, hope or fear, is the cause of an agitation whose influence extends to the heart."

It is now widely recognized that there are emotional and spiritual factors involved in creating and maintaining heart health. Books on women's health and midlife health in general emphasize the importance of "opening the heart at midlife." Leading heart specialists such as Dean Ornish, M.D., and Mehmet Oz, M.D., also ask us to consider that unresolved emotional and spiritual issues, such as a broken heart, depression, anger or lack of fulfillment, can physically affect the health of the heart.

Christiane Northrup, M.D., an expert in women's and midlife health, describes the heart as "an organ whose functioning is enhanced by joy, appreciation and passion." In order to create heart health, she believes, we need to recognize and respond to six basic emotions: love, joy, anger, sadness, fear and shame. Dr. Northrup's thinking is in line with Drs. Ornish and Oz, who maintain that the vessel-constricting effects of

Each of us is called to individuate, though not all will hear or heed. If we do not tend to our own process, our own journey, we risk denying the life forces that led to our incarnation and losing our sense of meaning. As long as we are on the high seas of the soul anyway, why not be as conscious and courageous as possible?

—James Hollis,
The Middle Passage: From Misery to Meaning at Midlife

negative emotions will be minimized if you are able to feel these emotions fully and let them flow. Positive emotions, if allowed to flower fully, open the vessels, optimizing blood flow and nourishing your tissues.

Some women experience heart symptoms related to anxiety, fear and depression. Learning to work with your emotions allows you to live fully, communicate with others and be motivated to make essential changes in your life. A healthy cardiovascular system is inextricably related to the free expression of joy and creativity.

Yoga's system of healing the heart aims to remove the obstacles to a healthy heart and circulatory system and allows the body to function as naturally as possible. Yoga philosophy recognizes that the heart-center is the seat of our truest connection with ourselves. It is the place where body, mind and spirit all converge. Many practitioners, including myself, experience feeling the heart-center open, feeling the sun in the heart-center radiate. Yoga practice often brings a physical, emotional and spiritual experience of one's inner happiness returning, although it would be more accurate, perhaps, to describe it as uncovering one's inner happiness. In other words, the parting of the clouds causes the sun to reappear—it does not cause it to shine more brightly.

Stress, Yoga and the Heart

Stress is now considered a significant contributor to poor health and an important factor in the development of heart disease, cancer and many chronic and acute diseases. Most modern-day stress reduction techniques have their roots in yoga and its emphasis on the breath and deep relaxation.

Cutting-edge health researcher Herbert Benson, M.D., first coined the phrase "relaxation response" in the 1970s to describe the profound physical and mental responses that occur when we consciously relax. Benson was the first among a growing number of scientists to document yoga's ability to significantly reduce stress, improve health and benefit the heart.

The practice of yoga encourages us to *observe* our reactions to daily events. Through the process of self-observation, we become aware of the totality of our responses to emotions such as fear, anger and anxiety. When we are angry or anxious, our whole being is involved. The breath becomes rapid and shallow to provide us with more oxygen to "do battle" or run away. The muscles begin to contract. Our metabolism and heart rate speed up, boosting strength and energy. The amount of blood pumped with each heartbeat increases. All this is nature's way of preparing us to attack a "predator" or protect ourselves.

The next time you feel angry, try to feel how your digestive system begins to shut down so that blood and energy can be diverted to the large muscles needed for fighting or running. If you are really angry, the arteries in your arms and legs will begin to constrict, and your blood chemistry will change so that clots form more quickly to conserve your blood should you be wounded.

I know no better
definition of life than
Jung's that "life is
a luminous pause
between two great
mysteries that yet
are one."
—James Hollis,
*The Middle Passage:
From Misery to
Meaning at Midlife*

Heart Palpitations

Many women experience a rapid or irregular heart-beat during perimenopause and menopause. Heart palpitations, often associated with hot flashes, can range from mild to severe and don't necessarily mean you are having a heart attack. Though rarely life threatening, they can be alarming. Their immediate cause is an imbalance between the sympathetic and parasympathetic nervous systems, which may result from unconscious fear and anxiety. If you have specific concerns about heart palpitations, see your health-care practitioner for further information.

According to heart and stress specialists, our bodies are designed to cope with acute stress, not the chronic stresses of modern life. When our survival mechanisms are activated chronically, they begin to exhaust our internal organs and nervous system. Arteries constrict not only in the arms and legs but also in the heart and brain. Blood clots are more likely to form inside the coronary and cerebral arteries, increasing blood pressure and sometimes leading to a heart attack or stroke.

Breathe Freely and Relax Deeply to Reduce Stress

Taking time to deeply relax and reduce stress is not a luxury but a health-promoting and potentially life-extending technique. The breath is the bridge between the body and mind. Our heartbeat responds to our breathing pattern. It gently accelerates when we inhale and slows when we exhale. The emphasis in yoga on inhaling slowly, gently, without strain and exhaling completely is relaxing for the heart muscle. Quick, shallow, upper chest breathing stimulates the sympathetic nervous system (which governs the stress response) and raises the heart rate and blood pressure in preparation for quick action. When our exhalations are longer, the parasympathetic nervous system (which governs the relaxation response) takes over, lowering the heart rate and blood pressure. Begin now to become aware of your breath and take time to practice slow, gentle, calm, even breathing. It's the first step to feeling more relaxed.

Posture Also Affects the Health of Your Heart

Our everyday posture—the way we sit, stand and walk—affects our respiration, circulation and the health of the heart. Chronic slouching decreases circulation to all the vital organs.

When your chest is collapsed, the diaphragm barely moves down as you inhale. This keeps you from filling your lungs completely. It prevents the "chest pump" from helping to return blood to the heart. If the abdomen and chest are compressed most of the time, the lymphatic vessels, arteries and veins serving the vital abdominal organs may be constricted or even collapse. This reduces the circulatory cleansing of these tissues, minimizes the transport of vital nourishment to the cells and interferes with the distribution of important hormones that regulate the body's processes. All this compromises the overall health of the body, including the heart.

One of yoga's most immediate effects is improvement in our posture. The body almost sighs with relief as the chest opens and the breath flows freely. Standing poses, backbends and inverted poses open the chest and expand the breathing process. Upward and Downward Dog, both from the floor and with the aid of wall ropes, stretch the muscles of the front of the body, expand the chest, increase breathing capacity, and strengthen the back, chest and shoulder muscles.

Gentle supported backbends and various restorative postures expand the chest, lungs and rib cage without effort. These passive poses are useful for everyone, but are especially recommended after healing from heart surgery. They should be practiced with the guidance of a qualified instructor.

Krishna Raman, M.D., a leading expert and writer on the integration of yoga with Western medicine states:

Backbends are particularly important for preventing and relieving coronary problems. This holds good even for the menopausal woman. Forward bends with support relieve elevated blood pressure. Inversions are very important to enhance and maintain a healthy circulatory status. They preserve the integrity of the facial tissues and relieve stagnation of fluid in the legs. They also prevent generalized water retention during the menstrual cycle by regularizing the hypothalamic-pituitary axis, which regulates water balance in the body. Inversions give rest to the heart from the strain of gravity.

All standing poses are useful for increasing circulation in the heart and throughout the body. Lying Down Hero Pose, Supported Bridge Pose and backbends such as Lying Back Over a Chair and Upward-Facing Bow *(Urdhva Dhanurasana)* are among the postures most noted for their effect on the health of the heart.

Without adequate physical activity, our circulatory system becomes sluggish. Constant standing increases stress on the veins of the legs, causing varicose veins. Many women suffer swollen feet at the end of the day due to poor return of body fluids to the heart. This circulatory problem is aggravated during the menstrual cycle when some women complain of leaden feet and a heavy feeling throughout the body. This is due in part to fluid retention owing to hormonal changes. Yoga's inverted poses are one antidote to this common problem.

Under conditions of intense chronic stress, even the muscle fibers inside the heart itself can begin to contract so vigorously that the normal architecture of these fibers is disrupted, damaging the heart muscle. To me this is an amazing metaphor: The inability of the heart to relax causes the heart's muscle fibers to constrict to the point that it damages itself— like clenching your fist so hard and for so long that the bones and knuckles in your hand begin to break.
—Dean Ornish, M.D.

High Blood Pressure (Hypertension)

Nearly 20 percent of adults in the United States have high blood pressure (hypertension). Hypertension is caused by multiple factors, including improper diet, stress, lack of exercise and excess body fat. It increases the risk of not only hardening of the arteries and heart attacks, but also ministrokes in the brain, which may result in dementia.

Restorative Yoga Poses known for relieving heart palpitations and breathlessness, regulating blood pressure and calming the nervous system include Supported Deep Relaxation Pose, Supported Lying Down Bound Angle Pose, Supported Standing Forward Bend Pose, Supported Downward-Facing Dog Pose, Supported Child's Pose, Supported Seated Forward Bends, Supported Legs Up the Wall Pose and Supported Bridge Pose.

Daily stretching, supported inverted and backbend poses and deep relaxation and meditation are crucial for the heart health of menopausal women. Inverted poses improve circulation, especially in the legs, increase blood flow to all the regulatory centers of the body and help control blood pressure.

Yoga postures also help maintain the elasticity of blood vessels. Passive backbends stretch cardiac vessels. Yoga breathing practices help prevent rhythm disturbances of the heart. Standing poses strengthen cardiac reserves. Forward bends improve the function of the sympathetic nervous system, which in turn affects cardiac nerves. Backbends force the heart to contract, lengthening cardiac muscle and enhancing blood flow.

Facts About Heart Disease for Women*

- Heart disease is the number one killer of women.
- One out of every two women will die from heart disease.
- Heart disease kills six times more women than breast cancer each year, and more than all other cancers combined.
- One in ten women age forty-five to sixty-four already suffers from some form of heart disease.

A Note to Teachers, Doctors and Other Health Professionals: See the Resources section for Yoga of the Heart Cardiac Teacher Training with Nischala Joy Devi and further information on yoga research and heart health.

Source: The National Coalition for Women with Heart Disease.
www.womenheart.org

Recommended Reading

A Matter of Health, by Dr. Krishna Raman (see chapter on Yoga and Cardiovascular Disorders)

Yoga Rx, by Larry Payne, Ph.D., and Richard Usatine, M.D. (see chapter on The Circulatory System: High Blood Pressure, Heart Disease)

Key Poses for Heart Health and High Blood Pressure

See chapter 8, "Yoga and the Wisdom of Menopause Practice Guide," for instructions.

Reminder: Do not be in a hurry. Select only the number of poses you can do without feeling rushed. **Time suggested is the minimum time.** Experienced practitioners can stay in poses longer.

Pose	Suggested Time
Supported Deep Relaxation Pose	10 minutes
Supported Lying Down Bound Angle Pose	10 minutes
Wide Angle Standing Forward Bend with Head Supported	1 minute or longer
Standing Forward Bend with Head Supported	1 minute or longer
Supported Downward-Facing Dog Pose	1 minute or longer
Hanging Downward-Facing Dog Pose	1 minute or longer
Supported Lying Down Hero Pose	5 minutes
Lying Back Over a Chair or Backbender	1 minute or longer— length of time according to experience and comfort
Supported Legs Up the Wall Pose	10 minutes
Supported Bridge Pose	5 to 10 minutes
Deep Relaxation Pose with Bolster Under Legs, Sandbag Across Abdomen	5 to 10 minutes

Virginia Lee, age 47

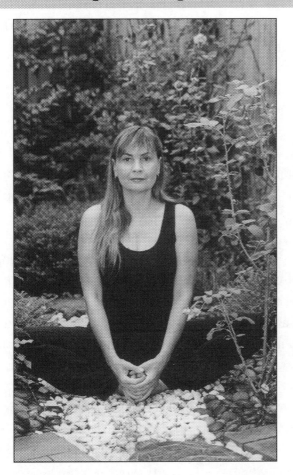

A Time for Moving into the Wisdom of Cronehood

My menopause experience has been a profound journey of healing and self-discovery. It is said that menopause is one of the most powerful times in a woman's life. I believe menopause is a doorway to true inner wisdom.

The first symptoms came early—about age forty-three—and included irregular periods, hot flashes, mood swings and depression. Because I was so young, I was unsure at first what was happening. I am now forty-seven and haven't had a period for two years.

Unfortunately, I did not have the benefit of the experience and wisdom of elder women in my family. My mother, her sister and my grandmothers all had hysterectomies and were on hormone replacement therapy. No matriarchs in my family went through natural menopause.

What got me through the intensity of my symptoms was a deep inner knowing that my body had the capacity to do this on its own. I knew that I came equipped with everything I needed to move through menopause, although the symptoms were uncomfortable. I believed that all I had to do was listen to and trust my body's wisdom and I would be all right.

At the time my menopausal symptoms first started, I had just begun teaching at the Southern California Woman's Herbal Symposium, a yearly event where nearly ninety women come together to educate and nurture one another and just be together. There I took a class on herbal remedies for menopause. The class confirmed that I was indeed menopausal, that my symptoms were normal and that there were many natural ways to treat the symptoms. I learned about Vitex, pomegranate juice (a powerful phytoestrogen), the herb dong quai and dietary considerations. I began to track

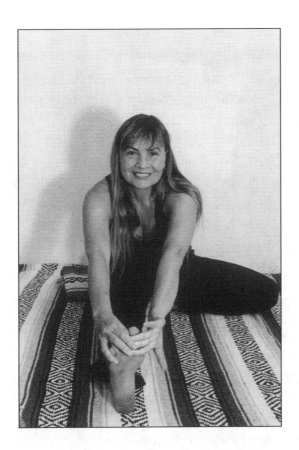

what I ate before getting a hot flash. Chocolate, for instance, would give me a powerful hot flash within about twenty minutes.

I found comfort and solace in my older women friends who had gone through menopause naturally and gracefully. One of the most helpful statements was from a friend who referred to hot flashes as "power surges." I came to experience hot flashes as my body deeply detoxifying itself. My body had its own wisdom, and I realized I did not need a physician to go through menopause. I was going through one of the most powerful times in my life, a time of deepening and moving into the wisdom of cronehood. I was actually proud to be going through it at such a young age, and I was determined to change the stereotype of what a menopausal woman was—old and dried up. I wanted to show the world that it could be done gracefully, that I could still be vital, fit, flexible and youthful—with wisdom to boot!

Part of staying vital was my yoga practice. I truly believe that yoga is one of the secrets to gracefully aging and is of utmost importance in regulating menopausal symptoms.

At the time my symptoms started, I was attending more rigorous Astanga classes, but during my symptomatic times, I was drawn back to an Iyengar style. I needed the precision and depth that this therapeutic method offered. I joined Suza's classes, with mainly midlife and older women, and the pace of the class was perfect for my needs. We went deeply into the poses and held them long enough for my body to really let go.

I also felt a deep sense of community with many women in the class who were my age and older, who had also transcended the stereotypic ideals of what older women are supposed to be like. These women were vital and flexible and have since become my role models. I feel it is extremely important to have role models of older women who have come through menopause, take care of themselves, stay healthy and age gracefully.

One of my greatest teachers during this time was the depression that accompanied menopause. As I learned to be with my depression, rather than struggle against it, I learned how to go deeper into myself. The depression was a voice inside me clamoring to be heard, a voice that had been ignored for a long time. Rather than medicate, I chose to honor and listen. The depression, along with a strong desire for time alone and with nature, led me to go on vision quests—searches to find the true nature of my being. That search has led me to deep and unconditional places of true peace within.

My sexuality has also deepened through menopause. My libido went through a change, but with that change was a deepening of my viewpoint on sexuality. Instead of wanting sex for itself, I wanted deep connection and to be fully present with another. I did not see the decreased libido as something bad or wrong, I saw it as an opportunity to continue to deepen spiritually and to bring that spirituality into the bedroom.

What also changed was the superficial way in which I had identified myself as a sexy woman. I gained about ten pounds, which challenged me to love myself in a way that is deeper than how I look. I realized that much of my self-esteem was contingent on looking like what our youth-oriented society feels is beautiful. I have come to reconciliation within myself: yes, I am aging, but my beauty comes from a much deeper place than outward appearance.

Menopause has been a time to discover myself and find what is true for me. I am learning how to accept and love myself in deep ways. I am rediscovering my connection with nature, other women and my body. I feel it is a blessing, not a curse, and is something to be truly honored in our own lives and in the women who have come before us. I have a strong desire to bring back the ideal of the crone, the elder woman that our youth can come to for wise counsel.

Virginia Lee is a life coach for health and well-being, massage therapist and yoga teacher. She also helps lead retreats for women with her spiritual teacher, Neelam.

Denise Lampron, age 50

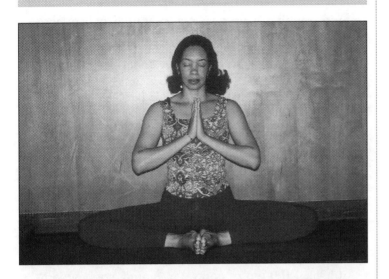

Menopause as a Spiritual Gateway

My introduction to yoga coincided with the commencement of my first moon cycle.[1] As a very flexible twelve-year-old, I effortlessly assumed the Full Lotus Pose *(Padmasana)* and was able to practice yoga poses with ease. Entering menopause would challenge everything I had previously called "truth," leaving me to rely on yoga and on the spiritual heritage of my stepfather and Native American great-grandmother.

Because of fibroid tumors, I had a partial hysterectomy in my early thirties, which officially ended my moontime. With one ovary remaining,

[1] *Native American tradition refers to the menstrual cycle as "moontime" because of the correlation between a woman's menstrual cycle and the twenty-eight-day cycle of the moon.*

however, I continued to ovulate during the full moon, which was the same pattern I had experienced before my partial hysterectomy.

Fifteen years later I entered menopause. It was July and the heat of summer felt particularly oppressive. The sun was no longer dancing off my skin and warming my body externally. The heat felt internal. It was surging up from deep inside my body and bursting outward, volcano-like. Uncontrollable torrents of water would cover my face, my scalp, my neck, under my arms and around my belly. A thin layer of perspiration dampened my forearms and legs. With each unsolicited explosion of heat, I felt out of control, a feeling soon accompanied by a sense of melancholy.

One Friday morning, I was sitting under the hairdryer at a local salon next to a friendly older woman who noticed my profuse perspiration. I *casually* mentioned my symptoms. The look of understanding, compassion and experience that bounced from her eyes to my soul exposed to me my own denial. I wept silently for six months. Finally, I accepted I was in menopause. I was old. I was undesirable. I was a crone.

Periods of crashing fatigue prohibited a rigorous yoga practice. I relied on various forms of breathing exercises *(pranayama)* and on gentle, relaxing poses when I couldn't sleep. I practiced restorative poses from Judith Lasater's book, *Relax and Renew,* when I needed to feel physically and emotionally supported.

My inner rhythms were different from anything I had ever experienced before. I desired to create a foundation upon which these new rhythms could thrive—a foundation that went beyond my body. Since menopause mirrors adolescence, it was time for maturing physically and emotionally. I uncovered aspects of my personality that still expressed the seventeen-year-old maiden. I embraced those aspects and encouraged them to join me in my current fifty-year-old body and life.

I craved the company of nature with its nurturing abilities. I practiced yoga on my patio, on the rooftop of my apartment building, during the full moon, at the beach and in the desert. Sometimes I simply sat in comfortable cross-legged poses and let my body touch the earth. Other times I practiced Deep Relaxation *(Savasana)*, also called Corpse Pose, under the light of a full moon. On days when I felt stronger, I would complete several rounds of Sun Salutations balanced with other poses that felt appropriate.

In the evening, after a particularly stressful day (the more stress—the more hot flashes), I would practice Legs Up the Wall Pose, which was extremely relaxing and brought blood and circulation to my legs and pelvic center. This pose also calmed my nervous system, allowing better sleep. The melancholy was greatly relieved after several months of practicing a gentler variation of Headstand. I relied on Supported Headstand during the summer, as a full, weight-bearing Headstand produced too much heat in my body.

I began to breathe *with* my hot flashes and to experience them as power surges or Kundalini[2] rising within my body. A yielding quality developed within my practice, replacing a more forceful attitude. This new approach to yoga was ideal during my change. Slowly my body began to stabilize and I felt stronger. During the summer I practiced in the morning, the coolest part of the day, and refrained from too many backbends or heat-building postures while incorporating the *sheetali* breath[3] which cools the body. Each day began with a prayer (talking to God/Goddess) and each evening ended with a meditation (listening to God/Goddess). Surrendering was sweet.

I supported my regular yoga practice with massage, acupuncture, chiropractic adjustments, craniosacral treatments, and belly and tantric dance[4] classes.

With continued awareness of my body, I could feel the constriction that was in my chest, and I began practicing chest-opening postures along with a daily meditation to release stale emotions and feelings lodged in my heart. This process required that I address my childhood patterns of not expressing my

---

[2] *Kundalini is a mythical Hindu serpent goddess who is said to lie asleep at the base of the spine. Under certain circumstances, including yoga and meditation, she rises through the body—in the form of powerful energy—to the top of the head.*

[3] *To practice sheetali breathing, curl your tongue, inhale, close your mouth and exhale normally through the nose.*

[4] *Tantric dance allows the experience and feelings of our sexuality to inspire our bodies to dance. This form of dance is extremely liberating and enhances sexual self-esteem while promoting graceful movement.*

feelings at the time that I experienced them. I wrote letters to parents, family, friends, employers and coworkers, and imagined them standing in front of me as I read the letter aloud. I then burned the letter. I began to understand how to feel the emotion, but not let it get stuck in my body. I created enough space in my chest for my heart to finally begin opening up. Chest-opening poses, which previously were painful, were now a pleasure to practice!

I began teaching a Full Moon Yoga class in order to give other women and myself the opportunity to gather at the time of the full moon, a potent moment for expression, dance and celebration. The class was an occasion to practice yoga, discuss spiritual issues and experience the power of being in a circle of supportive women. We did fire ceremonies (dances of passion around a blazing fire, symbolically throwing our past into the flames); Earth ceremonies (expressing gratitude to Mother Earth in the form of reading poetry, planting seeds and flowers, chanting together in praise of Earth); water ceremonies (yoga postures to enhance sexuality and sensation in the body, bathing in a stream or backyard pool, tantric dance); and completion ceremonies (honoring deaths, acknowledging ended marriages/relationships and lost jobs).

I created Yoga and Menopause workshops to teach postures that support women throughout menopause, to share my experience of diminishing symptoms while practicing yoga and to apprise women of the meaning of this powerful and important time in their lives. This is the first time many women have focused on their uterus for purposes other than childbearing. Poses increasing pelvic strength for greater sexual sensitivity and satisfaction are discussed and practiced. Bridge Pose is done with the intention of toning the reproductive tract and giving a woman greater pelvic motion. The Goddess Pose (Lying Down Bound Angle Pose) allows for an awareness of the vaginal canal and uterus, while other poses are beneficial stretches for the breasts. Downward-Facing Dog Pose and Squatting are both good poses for the bones in the legs. Partial and full inverted poses bring blood to the brain and to the pituitary gland, which controls hormone levels and is associated with the state of bliss.

The Native American tradition speaks of "moonpause" as being the most powerful time of a woman's life. It is a time of reflection and redirection. Our inner vision is expanded, our knowledge springs forth from the deepest part of our being and we are capable of extraordinary creativity. It is the pause between where we have been and where we are going. Our soul is seeking our attention.

My spiritual growth accelerated after I entered menopause. My intellect and ego took a backseat to intuition and inspiration (spirit in the body). Some experiences left me physically and emotionally exhausted, others left me joyful. All were necessary in the journey to wise woman. Hatha yoga provided the physical foundation my body required, while breathing *(pranayama)*, meditation and nature supported my sense of well-being.

Yoga and dance have become my soul mates. Together they have encouraged my body to stretch beyond past boundaries, to detach from my emotions, to melt my inhibitions and to follow my urges. They set my "wild woman" free, which is crucial to my creativity. Tying my pants or wrapping my skirt below my belly button when dancing, practicing yoga or relaxing at home, reminds me to celebrate the female roundness of my belly. Studying tantra has helped me reclaim my feminine nature, appreciate my sexuality and transform the feelings of being less desirable as I age. I no longer feel old; I am healthy and wise.

Over the years, I have seen yoga escalate from a "hippie exercise" of the 1960s to a structured science of the twenty-first century. After many years and countless classes, yoga remains not just a physical workout but a spiritual stepping-stone for me.

To every Wise Woman—walk in beauty.

Denise Lampron is a certified yoga teacher and wellness educator who developed Menopause as Spiritual Gateway—*a workshop for women already in menopause who desire a deeper understanding of the spiritual aspects of menopause.*

8 Yoga and the Wisdom of Menopause Practice Guide

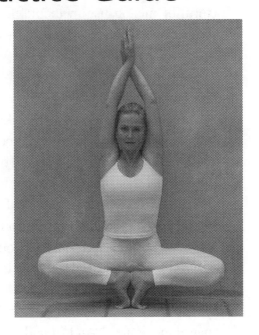

*The fate of the world is in our hands—
or, more accurately, in our minds and hearts.
As we begin to realize the creative effects of our
individual thoughts and emotions on collective events,
we will begin to use our God-given powers more
consciously and wisely—to build a better
world for all life on our beloved planet.*

—CORINNE MCLAUGHLIN, *SPIRITUAL POLITICS:
CHANGING THE WORLD FROM THE INSIDE OUT*

Yoga and the Wisdom of Menopause Practice Guide

Yoga has been used as a tool for physical, emotional and spiritual health for thousands of years. For women at midlife and beyond, yoga offers a primary form of menopause medicine that can help them cope with a wide range of symptoms without negative side effects. The yogic practices that support good health as a woman's body moves through menopause also help her make the most of her passage into the wisdom years.

No matter how tired or cranky I feel, even a short yoga session works wonders, especially when practiced with the help of props. In the world of yoga, a prop is any object that provides height, weight or support, and helps you stretch, strengthen, balance, relax or improve your body alignment. Props also help you stay in poses for a longer time and conserve your energy, allowing the nervous system to relax. This is especially important during menopause.

I tell my students that yoga bolsters are my "menopause medicine." "And," I add, "you will not hear about a study ten years from now saying bolsters are bad for you!"

The development of practicing yoga with the help of props is credited to B.K.S. Iyengar. His most recent book, *Yoga: The Path to Holistic Health,* illustrates the use of props to treat or prevent a wide range of ailments. Supporting the body with props opens the door to "restorative yoga," which not only allows you to exercise the body without exerting any effort, but simultaneously relaxes and re-energizes the body. This is critical during times like menopause, when women often find themselves in a vicious cycle of feeling "too tired to exercise," and then feeling even more tired because they are *not* exercising.

Judith Lasater's classic, *Relax and Renew: Restful Yoga for Stressful Times,* is an excellent companion for exploring restorative yoga in more depth. I also highly recommend *The Woman's Book of Yoga & Health: A Lifelong Guide to Wellness,* by Linda Sparrowe and Patricia Walden, to deepen your understanding of how to use yoga for health problems that may occur at any stage of a woman's life but are beyond the scope of this book.

In the opening pages of this book, we acknowledged that women are cyclic beings whose lives are deeply affected by the ebb and flow of their hormones. We are part of nature, affected by the cycles of the moon and the seasons of the year. Menopause is a time when many women feel a longing to deepen their connection with nature, and to discover—or rediscover—the joy of practicing yoga in natural surroundings. We realize intuitively that being in nature helps us reconnect with our own nature. When I practice yoga outdoors, in nature, I truly experience my practice as a way to open to the divine.

The feminine path to self-realization unfolds when a woman reclaims her own authority over her body and her life. She learns to honor her own needs and rhythms, and to trust her body's innate wisdom.

Each day as you step onto your mat, make a decision to enjoy just where you are right now. Take a few moments, too, to contemplate how fortunate you are to be practicing this wonderful art. A casual glance at the morning paper is proof enough of the vast suffering, poverty, violence and homelessness that are the lot of so many human beings. If you are standing on a yoga mat and have time to practice even fifteen minutes, you are a fortunate person. If you have a yoga teacher, you have an invaluable gift and life tool available to very few people. In the spirit of this gratefulness, let your practice begin.
—Donna Farhi, *Yoga, Mind, Body & Spirit: A Return to Wholeness*

At some point after fifty, every woman crosses a threshold into the third phase of her life. As she enters this uncharted territory—one that is generally uncelebrated in popular culture—she can choose to mourn what has gone before, or she can embrace the juicy crone years.

—Jean Shinoda Bolen,
Goddesses in Older Women: Archetypes in Women Over Fifty

Perimenopause Yoga Practice Guidelines

To organize your practice around your monthly cycle, follow these general guidelines:

If you are still menstruating, your practice should be adjusted to your natural menstrual rhythm. The days of menstruation are generally experienced as a time of lower energy and feeling the need for self-nurturing and moving inward. Your yoga practice should support this need and focus on more quiet, supported, lying down restorative poses and supported forward bends. Practice restful poses in a peaceful, unhurried way.

During the three or four days immediately following your period, you can focus more on inverted poses—according to your ability to practice safely—to help balance and adjust your hormones. Geeta Iyengar and longtime teachers who have studied with her caution against jumping right into a vigorous practice immediately after menstruation. Mid-cycle is generally the best time for more vigorous and challenging poses, such as deep backbends and advanced variations in inverted poses.

Backbends and inverted poses are recommended between menstrual cycles. If you are skipping periods, have stopped your periods, or are officially post-menopausal, these principles of paying attention to your body's energy level still apply. It makes sense that poses of great exertion which require you to draw upon your energy reserves are not recommended if you feel depleted.

Yoga Props—An Investment in Your Health

Here are descriptions of the most frequently utilized props:

Yoga Bolsters

Yoga bolsters come in various shapes and sizes. They conveniently provide the support needed to stretch and relax deeply in the essential menopause restorative poses that follow. While firm blankets can substitute for bolsters if necessary, I highly recommend purchasing two large, firm bolsters from a yoga prop company or yoga center.

While the width and height of the yoga bolster may vary, what makes it effective is the fact that it provides a firm support for the entire length of your spinal column, from the lower back to your head, when you are lying down. The muscles of your abdomen, chest and back release their tension, lengthen and relax deeply.

Yoga bolsters are specifically designed so that the sides of your rib cage open and expand over the bolster and move downward toward the floor. When your rib cage expands laterally in this manner, your breathing capacity naturally deepens. The bolster leaves a vital, lasting impression on the body of what it feels like to have the chest open and free. Using the bolster enhances your awareness of your breath as well as your ability to regulate and deepen your inhalations and exhalations.

Note: Pillows or pieces of foam that the body sinks into do not have the same effect.

Eye Bags

Placing an eye bag (or eye pillow) over your eyes will help you relax more deeply. The eye bag's gentle

It's true, we do store some memory in the brain, but by far, the deeper, older messages are stored in the body and must be accessed through the body. Your body is your subconscious mind, and you can't heal it by talk alone.

—Candace B. Pert, Ph.D., *Molecules of Emotion: Why You Feel The Way You Do*

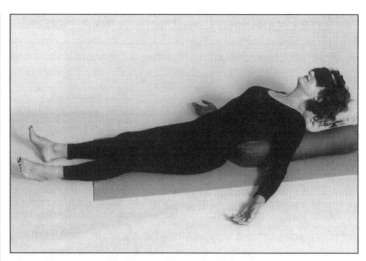

In Deep Relaxation Pose, the mind and body move inward, away from the surface of life. The mind and body become still. This state of peaceful awareness is the doorway to meditation.

pressure helps quiet the mind by relaxing the muscles around your eyes, calming the involuntary movements of your eyes, creating darkness and removing visual stimuli.

Sandbags

A yoga sandbag weighs ten pounds and is used to apply pressure to various areas of the body. A weight across the lower abdomen in Deep Relaxation Pose adds immensely to the depth of relaxation. When you first place the sandbag on your abdomen, you may be aware of the weight, but after about a minute your body accepts the weight and it seems to disappear. **Note:** Do not place a weight on your abdomen during menstruation.

Yoga Straps

A yoga strap is from six to ten feet long and is used in dozens of innovative ways in seated, lying down, inverted, standing and backbending poses. For some poses, like lying down leg stretches, you can substitute any soft belt or strap, but for most poses a real yoga strap with a buckle is much more convenient.

Yoga Blocks

Blocks are recommended for a wide variety of poses, especially for Standing Poses, where they support your hand if you feel strain attempting to reach the floor. They are also useful for seated poses, helping you to sit with your pelvis and spine in good alignment.

Yoga Mats

Last, but not least, if you don't already have one, do purchase a good quality sticky yoga mat. The beauty of a yoga mat is twofold: it provides a non-slippery surface, and it clears a space, both physically and psychologically, for you to do your practice. Many books and teachers recommend you make a space in your house to do yoga, or even dedicate an entire room. That is ideal, and I highly recommend it if you can do so. To my way of thinking, a dedicated yoga room is more important than a TV room or guestroom!

Keep your props in plain view so that they call to you to remind you to take time to stretch and relax—just like your toothbrush reminds you to brush your teeth. Think of your bolsters as furniture. When tired, get in the habit of lying down on your bolster instead of on the couch.

I believe it is through stillness and silence that the door opens. . . . Silence and solitude are the very basis for our engagement with the world.

—Joan Halifax,
The Fruitful Darkness

How the Poses in This Guide Are Organized

This Guide is divided into six main sections. The first section, especially recommended on days when you feel too tired to do anything else, consists of Essential Restorative Poses for crossing the menopausal bridge. I practiced these daily during the year that my periods stopped. The second section consists of Supported Downward-Facing Dog Pose and Supported Standing Forward Bends. The third section consists of other key weight-bearing Standing Poses to practice with the support of a wall or other prop. The fourth section consists of simple Seated Poses that can be integrated into your daily life, and two relaxing Lying Down Poses. The fifth section describes postures that require wall ropes or a backbender. The sixth section describes poses that are best learned under the guidance of a caring and knowledgeable teacher.

The poses described in this Guide provide a foundation on which to build a yoga practice that will help maintain your well-being during the menopausal years and beyond. All together they balance our fluctuating hormones and have a calming, soothing, quieting effect on the nervous system, thus helping to ease the menopausal symptoms described in this book.

Please note that most of these poses can be safely practiced on their own. For example, if you are feeling tired, practice Supported Legs Up the Wall Pose or Supported Lying Down Bound Angle Pose for ten minutes. If you have twenty minutes, practice both or stay in one pose longer. With practice, if you are patient and pay attention, your body will give you feedback on which poses you need most. Do not be in a hurry. Select only the number of poses you can do without feeling rushed. Think of your practice as an antidote to the rush-rush pace of modern life. It is far better to do fewer poses in a peaceful, leisurely way than to rush through too many.

There will be days when it is a blessing just to be still and rest deeply in one pose for as long as you like. It is always a good idea to end your practice with five minutes in Deep Relaxation Pose, either with the chest supported or a bolster under your legs, sandbag across your lower abdomen and eye bag over your eyes.

In all poses—and in all of life—keep your abdomen soft, your chest open and your breath flowing.

Section I: Essential Restorative Yoga Poses for Crossing the Menopausal Bridge

- **Supported Deep Relaxation Pose**—The pause that refreshes during "the pause" *(Supported Savasana)*
- **Supported Lying Down Bound Angle Pose**— The Goddess Pose *(Supta Baddha Konasana)*
- **Supported Child's Pose** *(Adho Mukha Virasana)*
- **Supported Bridge Pose**—The Menopausal Bridge Pose *(Setu Bandha Sarvangasana)*
- **Supported Legs Up the Wall Pose**—The Great Rejuvenator *(Viparita Karani)*
- **Deep Relaxation Pose** *(Savasana)* with bolster under legs, sandbag across abdomen, eyebag over eyes, legs straight or soles of the feet together on top of bolster

After a long stay in Restorative Poses, you will feel and look like you've had a massage and a facial. Your face and whole body will feel smoothed and soothed, from the inside out. Your eyes will look clearer and brighter. You will look at your world as if from the top of a mountain. The deep rest, peace and quiet you experience with restorative yoga is a doorway to meditation.

Note: Place your props for the following Restorative Poses on a sticky yoga mat or other non-slippery surface so they don't slide. If you have an eyebag, have it within reach so you can cover your eyes in the lying down poses. In cool weather, have an extra blanket handy for warmth.

Supported Deep Relaxation Pose—The Pause That Refreshes During the Pause (Supported Savasana)

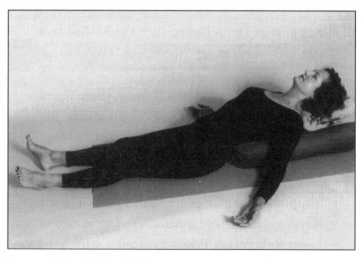

Supported Deep Relaxation Pose.

How to Practice: Sit in front of the bolster placed lengthwise behind you, with one or two folded blankets at the top to create a comfortable support for your head and neck. The edge of the bolster should touch your tailbone. Before lying all the way back, look down the front of your body and see if your upper and lower body are centered so that the line formed by your nose, chin, center of your chest, navel and pubic bone extends directly toward a center point between your heels.

Center your spine on the bolster. You may have to experiment with the height of the blanket under your head so that it feels truly comfortable. Your forehead should be slightly higher than your chin and not drop back.

Place an eyebag over your eyes. Relax your arms on the floor with your hands about a foot away from your hips. Turn your palms up and stretch your fingers outward, turning your thumbs toward the floor. Allow your arms and hands to soften and relax. Allow your legs and feet to relax and fall away from the midline. Your body should feel supremely comfortable, supported by the bolster, blankets and floor.

If you feel discomfort in your back, try repositioning your back on the bolster—you may be too high or too low on the bolster. Use your hands to move the flesh of the buttock down and away from your waist. If you still feel strain, decrease the height under your back.

Benefits: Practicing Deep Relaxation Pose on a bolster opens the chest and helps remove depression, as well as physical and mental fatigue. When we position our body on the bolster and lie still, we are practicing what yogis refer to as "deliberate stillness." Here we learn the art of deep relaxation. In Deep Relaxation Pose we experience divine rest. We give the mind and body a chance to integrate and also let go of the past. This pose is used to treat high blood pressure, relieve migraine and stress-related headaches, ease breathing problems and can be helpful for insomnia. If you have

Solitude. Blessed solitude has become very important to me. I find when I have a day alone, I just revel in it, bathe in it. It's the most incredible luxury. That seems to come with the fifties. Someone asked me, "Don't you get lonely?" I said, "I desire loneliness."
—Ellen Burstyn,
On Women Turning 50

Anything that is alive has to keep changing and keep evolving, and it's the same for yoga. The essence remains the same, but it has to keep coming out in different forms with each person who teaches it and with each generation.

—Angela Farmer,
Yoga Journal
July/August 00

trouble sleeping soundly, practice this pose before going to bed or if you cannot fall back asleep.

Note: You can practice Supported Deep Relaxation Pose for a few minutes and then move into the next pose, Supported Lying Down Bound Angle Pose. Or, you can begin your practice with Supported Lying Down Bound Angle Pose and move into Supported Deep Relaxation Pose by slowly straightening your legs.

Supported Lying Down Bound Angle Pose— The Goddess Pose *(Supta Baddha Konasana)*

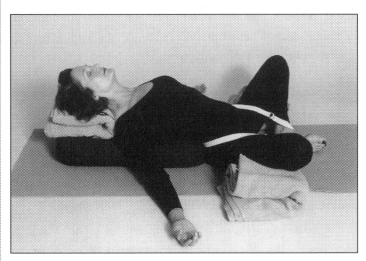

The Goddess Pose.

If you are new to this pose, you can skip the part of the instruction explaining how to strap yourself in. You can add the strap after you are more familiar with the pose.

How to Practice: Sit in front of the bolster placed lengthwise behind you, the soles of your feet together. As in Deep Relaxation Pose, have one or two folded blankets at the top to create a comfortable support for your head and neck. The edge of the bolster should touch your sacrum.

Loop a strap behind your back, at your sacrum (near your tailbone, not your waist). Bring it forward, around your hips, across your shins, and under your feet so that the soles of your feet are secure. Secure the strap in such a way that it is not too tight or too loose. (Ask your teacher to demonstrate this if you have not yet learned it in class.)

Center your spine on the bolster. Bring the soles of your feet close to your body. Place a folded blanket (or yoga block) under each of your outer thighs. The height of the blankets should adequately support the weight of your legs so that your back and knees relax. Your knees should be level. If one knee is much higher, place extra support under the lower knee. Many people also feel more relaxed with the support of a folded blanket under their forearms. Blankets can also be folded lengthwise and carefully positioned to support both the legs and arms.

Check that the height under your head feels comfortable. Place an eyebag over your eyes. Turn your palms up, allow your arms and hands to soften and relax.

As always, if you feel discomfort in your back, try repositioning your back on the bolster or try a smaller bolster or folded blankets. Or try increasing the height under your head slightly.

When you are comfortable, stay in the pose for ten minutes or longer. Observe the peaceful flow of your breath. To come out of the pose, place your hands under your thighs and bring your legs back together. Before sitting up, straighten your legs, allowing them to fall

Today's woman must be able to destroy any obsolete or irrelevant concepts that hobble her development. While nurturing her own inner life she does not neglect others, and she is careful to preserve all that is good in her present way of life. Such a woman is open to new perceptions that enable her to create new and more joyful ways of being. Activating her dormant powers, every woman can dance in eternal bliss on the corpse of her lesser self.

—Swami Muktananda Saraswati, B.A., *Nawa Yogini Tantra*

evenly away from the midline. When you feel ready, bend your knees, turn to your side, and use your hands to help you slowly sit up.

Benefits: Practicing Lying Down Bound Angle Pose with support from bolsters and blankets opens the chest, abdomen and pelvis and allows the body to relax deeply. Extra support under the forearms, knees and outer thighs makes the pose supremely comfortable and nourishing. Experts on yoga for women's health consider Lying Down Bound Angle Pose to be one of the most effective positions for regulating and balancing a woman's menstrual cycle and easing the symptoms associated with menopause. This supported position places the abdomen, uterus, ovaries and vagina in a position that frees these areas of constriction and tension that inhibit balanced hormonal activity. Blood flow is directed into the pelvis, bathing the reproductive organs and glands and helping to balance hormone function. The centering, balancing effect of this pose helps reduce mood swings and depression. This pose is also beneficial to those with high blood pressure, headaches and breathing problems.

Note: When you come out of Lying Down Bound Angle Pose, you can turn and face the bolster and relax in Supported Child's Pose.

Supported Child's Pose (Adho Mukha Virasana)

How to Practice: You will need a bolster or two blankets folded into the shape of a bolster. Sit on your heels with your knees on the floor, about hip-width apart. Place the bolster or folded blankets in front of you and lean forward until your torso and head are completely

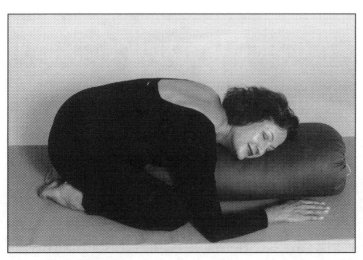

Supported Child's Pose.

Instead of always desperately struggling up somebody else's ladder, you have to thank them for what they gave you and then move on and climb your own.
—Angela Farmer,
Yoga Journal
July/August 00

supported. Turn your head to one side. Give yourself several minutes to relax and feel the soothing effect of the pose.

Remember to breathe softly, slowly, and truly "hug" your bolster. Allow yourself to sink into the bolster, relax and let go. Turn your head the opposite way before sitting up.

Benefits: For those moments when you feel like you're falling off the menopausal bridge and wish you could either stay in bed or run off and have a "crone's year alone," try retreating for a few minutes into Child's Pose. It gives you the opportunity to take a break and detach yourself from the sometimes seemingly impossible demands of life. This comforting, restful pose helps calm your nerves and emotions, helps lower blood pressure and feels wonderful on your back.

Note: You can practice Downward-Facing Dog Pose after Child's Pose, using the same support used in the previous poses to rest your head.

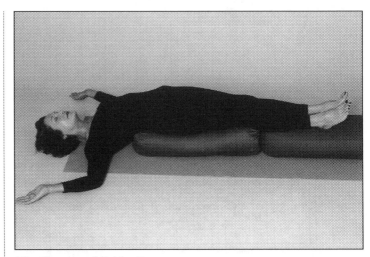

The Menopausal Bridge Pose.

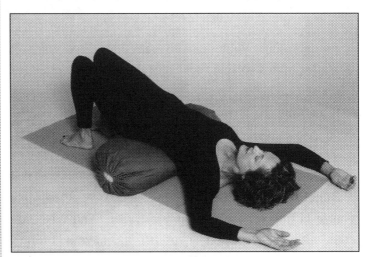

Gentle variation of the Menopausal Bridge Pose.

Supported Bridge Pose—The Menopausal Bridge Pose (*Setu Bandha Sarvangasana*)

Study the photo and note how the two bolsters under the back and legs are placed end-to-end to accommodate the length of the body. The height of the support depends on the length of your torso and the flexibility of your back. Taller people can add height to bolsters by placing one or more blankets on top of the bolsters. Make sure that your support is level.

How to Practice: Sit down on the bolsters, either with your legs straight out in front of you or with your feet on the floor on either side of the bolster. Position yourself near one end of the bolster so that when you lie down your head is near the far end. Use the support of your arms as you lie down. Slowly slide off the end until the back of your head and shoulders rest flat on the floor.

Observe how you feel. If you had difficulty lowering your shoulders to the floor, either use a lower support or place a folded blanket under your shoulders and head. If your lower back feels strain, try bending your knees and placing your feet on the floor on either side of the bolster. Relax your throat and chin. Lengthen and release your neck.

When you feel comfortable, close your eyes and cover them with an eye bag. Allow yourself to be still and listen to the beat of your heart. Allow your breath, mind and heart to slow down. Relax your arms out to the side at a comfortable angle, or with your elbows bent and arms relaxing back just above your shoulders (called "baby arms").

Stay in Supported Bridge Pose five or ten minutes or longer. When you feel ready to come out, remove your eye bag, bend your knees and slowly turn to your side. Or, you can slide off the bolster in the direction of your head, until your whole back and bottom are on the floor. Relax for a few more breaths with your lower legs supported by the height. Then bend your knees, turn to your side and slowly sit up.

Turn around, face the bolster, bend your knees, and briefly go back into Supported Child's Pose.

Benefits: Supported Bridge Pose is a combination gentle supported backbend and mild inverted position. You can clearly see and feel the opening of the chest and heart area as you place your body in this pose. It is restful for the heart and may help balance blood pressure and hormonal secretions. It has a calming effect on the mind and nervous system and helps prevent and relieve headaches. Placing your head lower than the rest of your body with the chest open is soothing and refreshing, and removes lethargy and depression. It also helps drain fluid from the legs after long periods of standing.

Supported Bridge Pose helps regulate and balance blood pressure. Women are more prone to elevated blood pressure when the protective effect of estrogen is withdrawn. When you stay in the pose, feel the effect deep inside the whole belly area. The effect of dropping the belly, uterus and ovaries in the pelvic bowl helps to balance the hormonal secretions and thus helps ease the hormonal fluctuations of menopause. This pose is recommended for relieving mood swings, hot flashes and tension headaches.

Supported Legs Up the Wall Pose— The Great Rejuvenator *(Viparita Karani)*

Have available two or three firm blankets or a yoga bolster. The blankets are placed under your bottom, which causes the rib cage to open and spread. The width of the blanket depends somewhat on your height and flexibility. For most people, the edge of the blanket can be placed at the waist. This placement allows the back

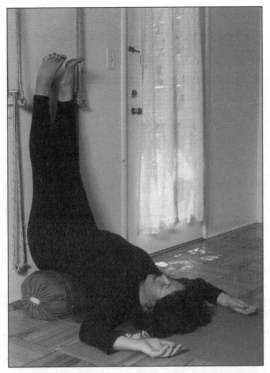

Supported Legs Up the Wall Pose (**Viparita Karani**).

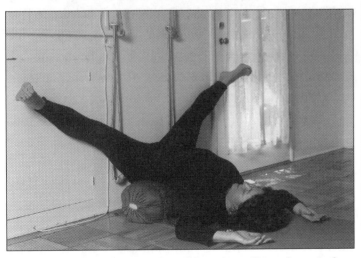

Variation of **Viparita Karani**. *One of the unique effects of yoga is the way in which the postures encourage blood flow through internal organs as well as the muscles.*

To recapture your *shakti-prana*, you must nurture a larger vision of who you are. You are not only an earthly mother, wife, daughter, sister, friend or career woman. You also live on the subtle plane of the spirit.

—Bri. Maya Tiwari,
*The Path of Practice:
A Woman's Book of
Ayurvedic Healing*

to curve in such a way that the lower lumbar spine is protected. The chest should appear and feel very open, so that the breath can flow freely.

How to Practice: Place a bolster about two or three inches away from the wall. Sit sideways so your right hip and side are touching the wall. With the bolster under your bottom, lower yourself back, using the support of your elbows and forearms, and swivel around to take your right leg and then your left leg up the wall. Keep your bottom as close to the wall as your leg flexibility allows. If you moved away from the wall and the bolster is not supporting your bottom and lower back, place your feet on the wall, lift your hips and move your bottom closer to the wall. If leg stiffness prevents you from being close to the wall, keep your bottom away from the wall, but pull the bolster toward you so that your lower back, lower ribs and bottom are comfortably supported by the bolster and your shoulders and head rest comfortably on the floor.

If you are new to yoga, you may find it helpful to first be familiar with simply relaxing with your legs on the wall. Sit on the floor beside a wall, knees bent, with one shoulder and hip touching the wall. Lower your torso toward the floor, keeping your bottom close to the wall, and swing around to bring your legs up the wall, supporting yourself on your elbows and forearms. Relax and lie back on the floor.

The next step is to lift your lower back off the floor and place a bolster or one or two folded blankets under your bottom, with your lower back supported. Experiment with the height of your blankets or bolster so that their support feels just right for your body—not too high or too low. If your neck or shoulders are uncomfortable, experiment with a small folded towel under the head or shoulders. The neck must feel comfortable, without any tightness or pinching at the nape. If blood flow to the head is obstructed, the brain cannot relax.

When you feel comfortable, close your eyes and cover them with an eye bag. Observe the rise and fall of your breath. Allow your heart and chest area to relax and open. Stay in the pose for ten minutes or longer.

Note: If you are tired, it is natural to fall asleep in this pose.

Follow Supported Legs Up the Wall Pose with a few minutes of gently stretching your legs on the wall before you slowly sit up. Stretch your inner thighs by slowly widening the legs, or practice a lying down variation of the Bound Angle Pose by bending your knees and bringing the soles of your feet together. Or, you can cross your ankles, allowing the wall to support your feet.

When you are ready to come out, bend your knees, turn to your side, and relax on the floor for a few more breaths before you slowly sit up. Follow with Child's Pose before moving on to the next pose. Finish your Restorative Yoga Practice with a few moments in Deep Relaxation Pose.

Benefits: Few things are easier and more refreshing, especially after standing upright for long periods of time, than simply lying on your back and elevating your legs up a wall or other surface. This is a safe and soothing way for women new to yoga to become accustomed to inverting their body. Practice this daily if your legs and feet swell easily, or if you have varicose veins.

During the year that my periods stopped, especially on hot days when the heat added to a sense of fatigue, I

Sadhana is a Sanskrit word whose root, *sadh,* means to reclaim that which is divine in us, our power to heal, serve, rejoice, and uplift the spirit. *Sadhana* practices encompass all our daily activities, from the simple to the sublime—from cooking a meal to exploring your inner self through meditation. The goal of *sadhana* is to enable you to recover your natural rhythms and realign your inner life and daily habits with the cycles of the universe. When you begin to live and move with the rhythms of nature, your mind becomes more lucid and more peaceful and your health improves. Your entire life becomes easier.

—Bri. Maya Tiwari, *The Path of Practice: A Woman's Book of Ayurvedic Healing*

practiced Supported Legs Up the Wall Pose for at least fifteen to twenty minutes every day, often much longer. I consider it among the greatest of yoga's inverted poses, because it safely inverts the body for long periods without any effort or strain on the neck.

This gentle inverted pose allows blood and lymph fluids to pool in the belly, soaking the reproductive organs in oxygen. It refreshes the heart and lungs, works to restore depleted energy and rebuild energy reserves. It is deeply relaxing during times of stress and tension and has a beneficial effect on the immune system. As you stay in the pose, the agitation and fatigue that accompany stress fade away.

Supported Legs Up the Wall is a gentle, inverted pose that can be practiced by almost everyone. It is a safe, non-threatening position that most people can hold long enough for gravity to return the blood from the extremities to the vital organs.

The way this restful, restorative yoga posture gently inverts the body without effort, it is almost physiologically impossible not to relax deeply. The "work" lies in learning how best to arrange your body. But once the body is in the right position, your job is to let go of all effort and just enjoy the feeling of relaxing.

Supported Legs Up the Wall is considered the most healing of the yoga restorative poses. When you turn upside down, gravity helps the venous blood—which otherwise tends to pool in the legs—to return easily to the heart. In people whose heart rates are elevated because they have not been receiving an ample supply of blood, this pose reduces the heart rate by improving the blood flow into the chest. In this gentle supported inversion, as in other more active inverted postures, the weight of the blood in the feet, legs and abdomen stimulates blood pressure receptors in the neck and chest to reduce the constriction of the arteries throughout the body. This reduces blood pressure.

Part of the soothing effect derived from Supported Legs Up the Wall is due to the angle of the torso. Note in the photo how the stack of blankets positioned under the pelvis brings the torso into a gentle supported backbend, while the wall supports the legs. As you lie in the pose, you can imagine that its shape creates an internal waterfall, as the fluid in the legs cascades down to the abdomen and spills over into the chest, toward the heart. This waterfall effect creates a peaceful, soothing sensation.

Cautions: People with heart problems, neck problems, eye pressure, retinal problems or hiatal hernia should use caution with all inverted poses. However, Supported Legs Up the Wall Pose is recommended for those with mild hypertension, because it can help normalize blood pressure. If you experience discomfort with your legs straight up the wall, experiment with helping your body become accustomed to the pose by first lying down with the lower legs resting on the seat of a chair or stool.

Deep Relaxation Pose with Bolster Under the Legs (Savasana)

How to Practice: Follow the instructions for Supported Deep Relaxation Pose but without the bolster under your back. Study the photo and note that in this variation of Deep Relaxation Pose, there is a bolster under the legs and a sandbag across the lower abdomen. You can practice as shown, with legs straight,

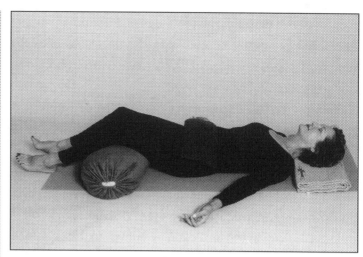

Deep Relaxation Pose.

or place the soles of the feet together as in Lying Down Bound Angle Pose, on top of bolster.

Place the bolster under your knees and lower yourself to the floor. Place a folded blanket under your head if that feels more comfortable. Stay in this pose for five minutes or longer. When you feel ready to sit up, bend your knees and turn to your side for a few breaths; use your hands to press the floor as you sit up.

Benefits: See benefits for Supported Deep Relaxation Pose. This pose relaxes the body, soothes the nervous system, lowers blood pressure and heart rate, and brings a sense of peace to the mind. Helps to relieve fatigue and insomnia.

Section II: Standing Forward Bends and Downward-Facing Dog Pose

- **Wide Angle Standing Forward Bend Pose with Head Supported** (*Prasaritta Padotanasana*)

- **Wide Angle Standing Forward Bend with Spine Concave, Head Looking Up**
- **Standing Forward Bend Pose with Head Supported on Chair** (*Uttanasana*)
- **Supported Downward-Facing Dog Pose** (*Adho Mukha Svanasana*)

Wide Angle Standing Forward Bend Pose with Head Supported *(Prasaritta Padotanasana)*

How to Practice: Place a chair with a folded blanket or bolster or other level support about two feet in front of you. Step your feet about four feet apart, heels a little wider apart than your toes. Keeping your legs straight by lifting up your front thigh muscles (quadriceps), bend slowly forward from your hip hinge. Adjust the height so

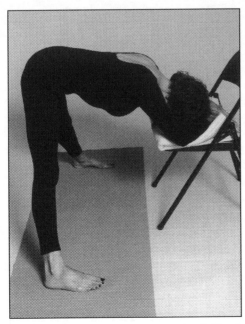

Wide Angle Standing Forward Bend with Head Supported on Chair.

that your head rests comfortably. Stay in Supported Wide Angle Forward Bend Pose for one to five minutes. To come up, place your hands on your legs and inhale deeply as you return to standing upright. Feel the calming, soothing effect of this pose.

Benefits: If your legs are very stiff, it is safer and more relaxing to bend forward with the feet wide apart. Resting your head on a chair as illustrated, or on a bolster or block, brings your head below the level of your heart and has a lovely cooling effect on your brain and nervous system. This calming effect may help ease hot flashes. As in other poses where the head hangs below the level of the heart, the pituitary gland (which regulates changes in hormone level) is stimulated.

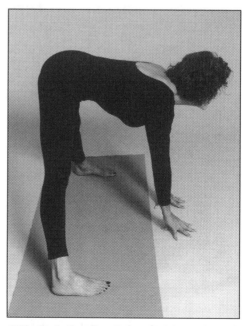

Wide Angle Standing Forward Bend with Spine Concave.

Wide Angle Standing Forward Bend Pose with Spine Concave, Head Looking Up

How to Practice: Step your feet about four feet apart, heels a little wider apart than your toes. Keeping the knees straight by lifting up the front thigh muscles (quadriceps), bend slowly forward from your hip hinge. Depending on your leg flexibility, place your fingertips or palms on the floor, block or other height, arms straight as illustrated, head looking up toward the ceiling.

Benefits: Helps lift and tone the uterus, improves circulation to the pelvis and may help ease heavy bleeding during perimenopause. Practiced with the spine concave, this pose strengthens the pelvic floor and prevents or relieves urinary incontinence.

Standing Forward Bend Pose with Head Supported on Chair (Uttanasana)

How to Practice: Place a chair with a folded blanket, bolster or other level support about two feet in front of you. Step your feet hip-width apart, heels a little wider apart then your toes. Keeping your legs straight by lifting up your front thigh muscles (quadriceps), bend slowly forward from your hip hinge. Adjust the height so that your head rests comfortably. Keep your legs straight by stretching up with your quadriceps muscles at the front of the thighs. You will see the definition of the front thigh muscles when you contract them. This action both stabilizes your knee joints and allows the hamstring muscles at the back of the thighs to release.

Stay in this Supported Standing Forward Bend for about a minute or longer. To come up, place your hands

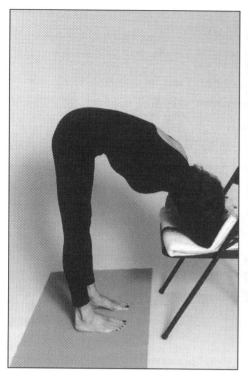

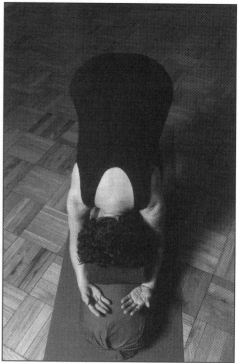

Standing Forward Bend with Head Supported.

Standing Forward Bend variation by a more flexible practitioner.

on your legs and inhale deeply as you return to standing upright. Feel the calming, soothing effect of this pose.

Benefits: This pose has many benefits similar to Wide Angle Standing Forward Bend Pose. It is a key pose for hormonal balance and heart health. It lifts the uterus and tones the pelvic floor. According to Geeta Iyengar, bending forward with a slightly concave back can help lift a prolapsed bladder or urethra.

Supported Downward-Facing Dog Pose
(Adho Mukha Svanasana)

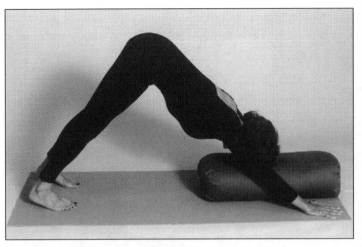

Supported Downward-Facing Dog Pose.

How to Practice: There are many different ways to come into Downward-Facing Dog Pose. When practiced after one of the other lying down supported poses, you can come to your hands and knees in front of the bolster. Place your hands on either side of the front edge of the bolster, fingers spread wide apart and in line. Bring your knees back in line with your hips. Place your feet hip-width apart, curl your toes under, press your hands firmly into the mat, push the floor away from you and, on an exhalation, straighten your legs so that your body forms the shape of an inverted V and looks like a dog stretching. Stretch back through your legs so that your hips move further back away from your hands. Stay high up on the balls of the feet until you feel your spine lengthening and abdomen lifting. Keeping the length in your spine, press your heels toward the floor. Allow your head to relax on the bolster. Do not strain to bring your head on the bolster. If your head does not touch, increase the height of your bolster with one or two folded blankets.

When you come down, separate your knees and come back to Supported Child's Pose.

Benefits: Downward-Facing Dog Pose inverts the internal organs and increases blood flow to the head. With the help of an experienced teacher, you can learn to use this pose to help lift and tone your uterus, improve circulation to your pelvis and strengthen your pelvic floor. It tones all the systems of the body, thus impacting the endocrine glands. It is a key pose for easing hot flashes. A weight-bearing pose for the upper body, it strengthens the bones in the hands, wrists, arms and shoulders, thus helping to prevent osteoporosis. Placing your head on the bolster as illustrated makes the pose more restful.

Note: Allow yourself at least one minute to relax in Child's Pose after Downward-Facing Dog Pose. Supported Downward-Facing Dog Pose can be practiced with the first series of Restorative Poses, as part of a sequence of Standing Poses or to prepare for Inverted Poses.

Section III: Supported Standing Poses

- **Supported Triangle Pose at the Wall** (*Utthita Trikonasana*)
- **Supported Warrior II Pose** (*Virabhadrasana II*)
- **Supported Extended Side Angle Pose** (*Utthita Parsvakonasana*)

- **Supported Half Moon Pose with Back to Wall, Windowsill or Counter** *(Ardha Chandrasana* with Back to the Wall)
- **Supported Half Moon Pose Facing the Wall** *(Ardha Chandrasana* Facing the Wall)

Standing poses safely remove the joint and muscle stiffness that many women experience during menopause and post-menopause. They also improve circulation and breathing, stimulate digestion, regulate the kidneys and relieve constipation. The back, hips, knees, neck and shoulders all gain strength and mobility with regular practice. Oxygen is drawn into the body, lifting feelings of lethargy and fatigue. The breath flows freely, and the whole body becomes energized.

Practicing Standing Poses either with your back to the wall or facing the wall conserves energy, improves body alignment, and increases the benefits during menopause. Depending on your height, about six feet of empty wall space is ideal. If wall space is not available, use a windowsill or kitchen counter. Many yoga centers have available a trestle (horse) shown in the photographs.

Triangle Pose, Warrior II Pose, Extended Side Angle Pose and Half Moon Pose are four basic standing poses that give the whole body a healthy tune-up and safely remove the heaviness and stiffness that tend to settle into the body when your periods stop.

Geeta Iyengar teaches that the best way to practice Standing Poses during menopause is with the front of the body facing a wall or trestle (horse). Do not contract or harden the abdomen. Focus on keeping your abdomen soft, passive and your chest open. Facing the wall lessens abdominal pressure and water retention. Half Moon Pose *(Ardha Chandrasana)* is most effective practiced at the wall (with the front or back of body supported by the wall). This pose is especially beneficial during menopause. It opens the pelvic and abdominal cavities and allows a healthy flow of oxygen to return. Half Moon Pose exercises the hip joint and is a key pose for strengthening the hips.

Caution: If you have osteoporosis, consult your teacher. Practicing with your back to the wall in this case may be more beneficial.

Supported Triangle Pose at the Wall or Other Support *(Trikonasana)*

How to practice: Stand tall with your posture open, shoulders relaxed, near a wall. Step your feet about four feet apart (depending on the length of your legs), keeping your feet/big toes in line, facing forward, heels close to the wall.

Anchor your feet to the earth by pressing the soles of your feet deep into the floor. Keep your legs straight by lifting up your thigh muscles. Allow your body to become taller and taller, lengthening your spine upward.

Raise your arms to shoulder level, palms facing down, and stretch out through your fingertips. Feel the center of your body expand and open. Breathe softly and smoothly.

When you feel stable and centered in this position, turn the left foot about 30 degrees in and the right foot 90 degrees out. Line up the right heel directly in line with the center of the left arch.

Inhale, and on exhalation stretch to the right from the hip joint, so that your torso stretches sideways as a unit

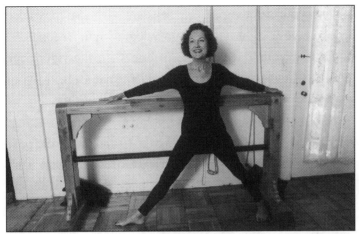

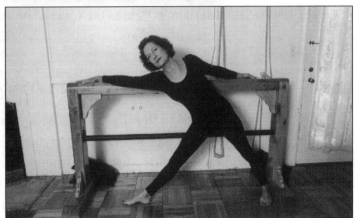

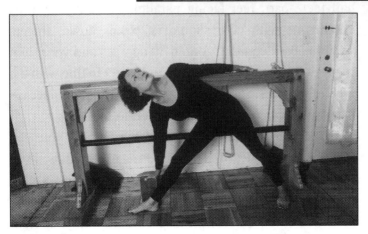

Supported Triangle Pose variation with arm on horse helps open the shoulder joint.

toward your right leg. If your legs are stiff, you may need to place your right hand on your leg, a chair or block.

Extend your left arm up, in line with the right arm, palm facing forward. If you feel unusual strain in your shoulder, try placing your left hand on your hip.

Stay in the pose for several breaths, keeping your legs straight, shoulders and neck relaxed. Come out of the pose on an inhalation, keeping your body close to the wall. Turn your feet to face forward. Relax back into the wall and pause for a moment to feel the effects of the pose.

Repeat on the other side.

Triangle Pose is the foundation for the three Standing Poses that follow.

Supported Warrior II Pose (Virabhadrasana II)

How to practice: Stand with your back against a wall and use the wall to help you maintain your awareness of good posture, just as in Triangle Pose. Keep your arms, shoulder blades and bottom in contact with the wall.

Separate your feet approximately four to four-and-a-half-feet apart, feet facing parallel. Stretch your arms out in line with your shoulders, palms down, fingers straight. Turn your left foot in 30 degrees and your right foot out 90 degrees. Keep your right heel in line with the arch of your left foot. Keep your legs straight, kneecaps lifted and both feet firmly anchored to the earth.

Exhale, and bend your right knee so that your leg forms a right angle. Stretch your arms in both directions, stretch your shoulders back and down, in contact with the wall or other support, to open your chest. Keep your abdomen lifted but soft, and gaze softly at your right hand. Keep your back leg straight and press both feet

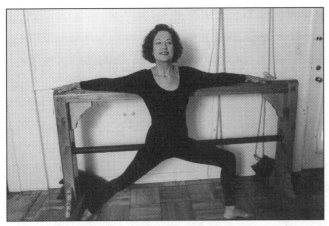

*Supported Warrior II Pose (***Virabhadrasana II***).*

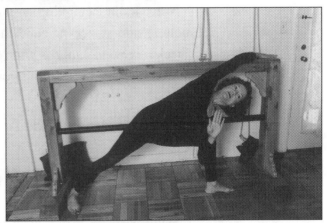

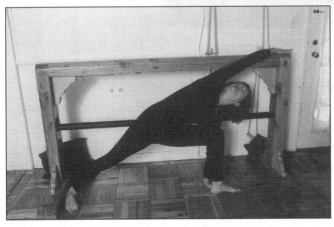

*Supported Extended Side Angle Pose (***Utthita Parsvakonasana***).*

strongly into the floor. Hold the pose long enough so that you feel your legs strengthening, but not so long that you collapse! Keep your breath flowing freely, lips closed softly.

To come out of the pose, straighten your right leg as you come up and turn your feet so they are back to the original parallel position. Turn your right foot slightly in and your left foot out 90 degrees. Repeat on the left side.

Benefits: Warrior Pose II strengthens the back and legs, develops strength and stamina and gives an intense stretch to the groins.

Note: In the beginning, you may not be ready to take such a wide stance or bend the knee to a right angle. Check that your stance is wide enough so that your bent knee is directly in line with your heel.

Supported Extended Side Angle Pose
(Utthita Parsvakonasana)

How to practice: Start with the same directions as in Warrior II Pose.

Stand with your back against a wall or other support and use the support to help you maintain your awareness of good posture, just as in Triangle Pose. Keep your arms, shoulder blades and buttock in contact with the support. Place a block within reach to the right of your mat.

Separate your feet about four feet apart, feet facing parallel. Stretch your arms out in line with your shoulders, palms down, fingers straight. Turn your left foot in 30 degrees and your right foot out 90 degrees. Keep your right heel in line with the arch of your left foot. Keep your legs straight, kneecaps lifted and both feet firmly anchored to the earth.

Exhale, and bend your right knee so that your thigh and calf form a right angle. Stretch your arms in both directions, stretch your shoulders back and down, holding onto the support of the trestle (horse) or a counter or windowsill; exhale and bend the right leg into a right angle, keeping your upper body in the center as much as possible and strongly anchoring through your back leg. Move into Extended Lateral Angle (Side Angle) Pose, lowering your fingertips to the floor or block. Beginners can place block in front of foot.

Supported Half Moon Pose (Ardha Chandrasana) with Back to Wall, Windowsill, Counter

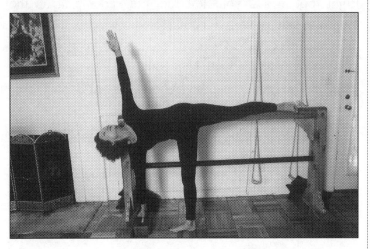

How to practice: Standing against the wall or other support, separate your feet four to four-and-a-half feet apart as in Extended Triangle Pose. Stretch your arms out in line with your shoulders. Turn your left foot slightly inward and right foot out 90 degrees, and, keeping the back of your head and both shoulders on the wall, come into Extended Triangle Pose. Slowly bend your right knee and place the fingertips of your right hand on a block, stool or chair seat, about a foot in front of your right foot.

Exhale and shift your weight forward and onto your right foot. Lift your left leg as your right leg straightens. Stay close to the wall so that when you move into the pose the back of your head, both shoulders, your whole back, both buttocks, your lifted leg and heel of the lifted foot all press back against the wall. Keep both legs straight. Lift your left arm toward the ceiling, palm facing forward. Turn your head as in Triangle Pose, and gaze at your left thumb. Keep your abdomen soft, pelvis and chest turning toward the ceiling.

Exhale back to Triangle Pose and inhale up. Turn your right foot in and your left foot out and repeat on the opposite side. When you complete both sides, it is cooling and relaxing to keep your feet wide apart. Move a little away from the wall, lean your hips into the wall and release slowly into Standing Wide Forward Bend Pose.

Supported Half Moon Pose Facing the Wall

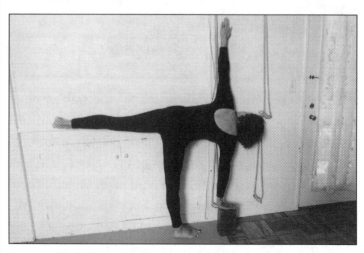

Supported Half Moon Pose Facing the Wall.

Practice the Half Moon Pose facing the wall or other support. In this variation, a wall works best.

How to practice: Stand facing the wall and step the feet about four feet apart as in Extended Triangle Pose. Come into Extended Triangle Pose with your arms in line with your shoulders but with the palms of your hands pressing the wall. Keep the front of your body as close to the wall as possible, pressing your palms into the wall continuously to help turn your chest and pelvic area to the ceiling.

Exhale and shift your weight forward and onto your right foot. Lift your left leg as your right leg straightens. Stay close to the wall so that when you move into the pose your face and upper body stay close to the wall. Your standing foot should remain turned out 90 degrees, a little away from the wall, but the toes of the lifted foot should brush the wall so that your lifted leg stays in line with your hip. Keep your abdomen soft, feel the opening in your pelvis, allow your breath to flow freely. Place your hand on a block (or even a low stool or chair seat) to reduce strain on your legs and to allow the pelvis and chest to open. Keep both legs straight. Lift your left arm toward the ceiling, palm facing forward, pressing into the wall to help open the chest and pelvis. Turn your head as in Triangle Pose, and gaze at your left thumb. Keep your abdomen soft, pelvis and chest turning toward the ceiling.

Exhale back to Triangle Pose and inhale up. Turn your right foot in and your left foot out and repeat on the opposite side. Practicing Half Moon Pose facing the wall is considered the most beneficial way to practice during menopause.

How long should you stay in Half Moon Pose and other Standing Poses? If you are new to yoga, twenty to thirty seconds, gradually increasing the length of time. I tell women in my classes to hold the pose long enough so they feel opened and strengthened, but not so long that they feel strain or fatigue. Even if you are a long-time practitioner who balances easily in the middle of the room, during menopause I highly recommend you allow yourself the luxury of practicing Standing Poses with support, with special emphasis on Half Moon Pose.

Benefits: Supported Half Moon Pose opens the pelvis and heart center, increases circulation, massages the organs of the abdomen and pelvis and may help relieve urinary tract infections in women. Practiced with the help of a wall, it may help slow or stop heavy bleeding and relieve cramping associated with fibroid tumors and endometriosis. Half Moon is excellent for lengthening the spine and strengthening your back, stretching the groins, opening the hips and strengthening the legs, ankles and feet. It also helps develop balance and coordination.

Practice Standing Wide Forward Bend in between all the Standing Poses to keep your body cool and tranquil.

Section IV: Important Seated and Lying Down Poses During Menopause

- **Seated Bound Angle Pose** *(Baddha Konasana)*
- **Seated Wide Angle Pose** *(Upavistha Konasana)*
- **Lying Down Big Toe Pose with Leg Opened Up to Side** *(Supta Padangusthasana II)*
- **Lying Down Bent Knee Twist** *(Jathara Parivartanasana)*

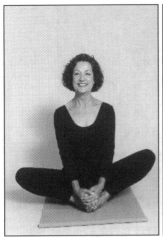 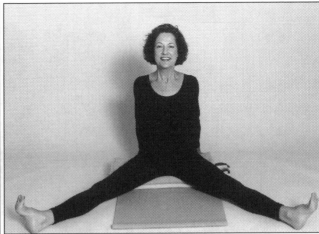

Seated Bound Angle Pose.   *Seated Wide Angle Pose.*

Seated Bound Angle Pose (Baddha Konasana)

How to Practice: Sit on one or two folded blankets or a yoga block. The height under your bottom depends on your hip flexibility. Bend your knees and bring your feet toward your pubic bone. Join the soles of your feet together. Place your finger tips behind your hips, lengthen your spine up toward the ceiling, lift and open your chest and press your legs toward the floor. A sandbag placed on your inner thighs, as illustrated, will help your thighs to relax. Keeping the lift in your spine, clasp your fingers around your feet. Keep your abdomen soft, face relaxed, breath flowing and allow your pelvis to open and groins to relax. Stay in the pose several minutes or longer.

Benefits: (See next pose)

Seated Wide Angle Pose (Upavistha Konasana)

How to Practice: Sit on the floor, on a folded blanket if necessary. Place the fingertips on the floor behind the

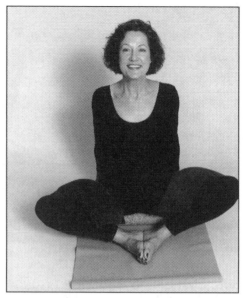

Seated Bound Angle Pose with sandbags on thighs.

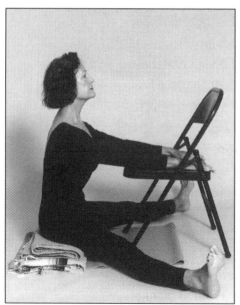

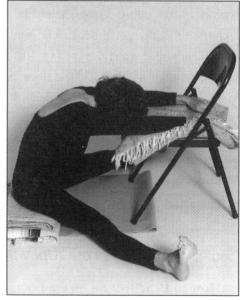

Sealed Wide Angle Pose using a chair opens the chest. Resting your head on a chair makes the pose more relaxing for beginners.

hips, and stretch your spine up. Check that your feet are an equal distance apart. Stay on the center of your heels and press the back of your legs into the floor. Relax your abdomen. Focus on opening and widening the pelvis.

Benefits: Bound Angle Pose and Seated Wide Angle Pose are two key sitting poses for easing a wide range of perimenopause and menopause symptoms. According to Geeta Iyengar, Bound Angle Pose tones the kidneys, alleviates urinary and uterine disorders, and strengthens the bladder and uterus. It eases menstrual problems such as cramps, heavy bleeding and heaviness in the abdomen. Seated Wide Angle Pose helps blood to circulate in and around the pelvic region, helps lift and tone your uterus, massages the organs of the reproductive system and stimulates the ovaries. Both these poses are calming and centering.

Lying Down Big Toe Pose with Leg Opened Up to Side (Supta Padangusthasana II)

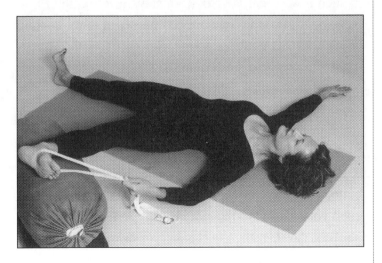

How to practice: Do the Lying Down Big Toe Pose and other lying-down poses with the props needed to allow you to practice in a way that feels restful deep inside your body. Lie on your back, both legs straight, feet together, upper and lower body in line. Place a bolster, two folded blankets, stool, block or other prop about a foot away from your right hip or foot. **Note:** The height and placement of the prop depends on your leg flexibility. Bend your right leg and loop a strap around the right foot, holding the strap with your right hand. Slowly straighten your right leg up to the ceiling, pulling the toes of both feet toward your body and extending through both heels. Think of making both legs longer and longer. With your right hand reaching up the strap, check that both legs are completely straight so that you feel the back of your lifted leg stretching. Keep your breath flowing, abdomen soft, face relaxed. Then, keeping the back of your body (both buttocks) firmly anchored to the floor, slowly open your right leg out to the side. Adjust the bolster or other support so that you can rest your leg in such a way that your bottom stays level on the floor. Relax in the pose for one or two minutes or longer—long enough so that you feel your abdomen and pelvis opening. Come back to the center and repeat on the left side.

In the beginning when you practice this pose, your mind will naturally be drawn to understanding the outer structure of the pose. The sensation of stretch at the backs of the legs may be overwhelming. There is also the muscular effort of keeping the body anchored—both buttocks firmly on the floor—when you first learn to open your leg out to the side. By supporting the leg with bolsters, stool, a stack of blankets or even a chair or sofa if the body is quite stiff, you will gradually go deeper inside your body and learn to relax your organs. Allow your abdomen, uterus and ovaries to remain soft.

Practicing in this way during menstruation encourages the blood to flow freely and relieves the feeling of congestion in the pelvis.

Practice this pose regularly to become familiar with the outer structure and alignment of the pose and the inner, healing effect on your internal organs.

Benefits: This is an excellent pose for relieving menstrual discomfort. It is beneficial for removing joint stiffness related to menopause and easing hot flashes. Lying Down Big Toe Pose II has many of the same benefits as Half Moon Pose and prepares your legs and hips for the more challenging weight bearing actions in Half Moon Pose.

Lying Down Bent Knee Twist—Gentle Floor Twist— Stomach Turning Pose (Jathara Parivartanasana)

How to practice: Lie down with your knees bent, feet flat on the floor, your upper and lower body in line. Place a folded blanket under your head if needed to keep your forehead and chin level so that your head does not tilt back. Bring your arms in line with your shoulders, palms up, hands actively stretching away from each other to open your chest. Allow your back to relax toward the floor.

Still keeping your feet flat, lift your hips up off the floor to move them gently to the left. Lower your hips back down. Bend your knees toward your chest, and slowly lower your knees to the right. **Note:** Be sure to use your abdominal muscles to lift and lower your legs. Do not just plop your knees to the floor. Lower with control.

Stretch your left arm away from your knees. Your right arm can stay in line with your shoulders, or you can increase the stretch by placing your right hand on your knees, gently pressing them down. Stay in this posture for a few breaths, allowing your body to release into the pose. When you feel ready, on an exhalation use your abdominal muscles to bring your knees back to the center. Move your hips to the right before slowly lowering your bent knees to the left.

Benefits: Gentle floor twists help prevent and relieve lower back pain caused by muscle tension. They also reduce cramps and indigestion and tone the abdominal area. The abdomen gets an internal massage in this pose. It also relieves tension and stiffness in the neck and shoulders.

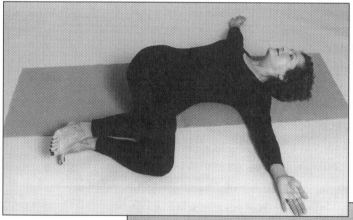

Lying Down Bent Knee Twist.

Variation.

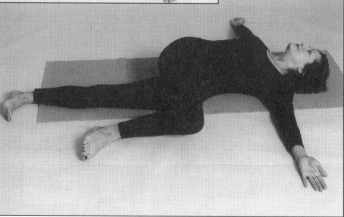

Note: If you feel back or shoulder strain, or if your knees cannot touch the floor, place a folded blanket under your knees.

More flexible students can practice Lying Down Bent Knee Twist Pose—with a bolster supporting their pelvis and mid-back—after doing Supported Legs Up the Wall Pose *(Viparita Karani)* or Shoulderstand.

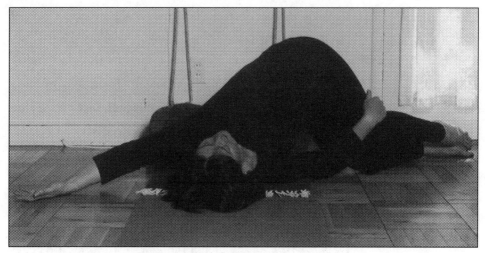

Lying Down Bent Knee Twist, bolster under bottom.

Section V: Poses Using Wall Ropes, Inversion Slings and Backbenders

- **Yoga Wall Ropes**—Another Investment in Your Health for Years to Come
- **Upward-Facing Dog with Wall Ropes**
- **Forward Bend with Wall Ropes**
- **Downward-Facing Dog Pose with Wall Ropes— Hanging Downward-Facing Dog Pose** *(Adho Mukha Svanasana)*

- **Supported Headstand Hanging from a Rope or Pelvic Sling** *(Sirsasana)*
- **Lying Back Over a Backbender** *(Viparita Dandasana* on a backbender*)*

Yoga Wall Ropes—Another Investment in Your Health for Years to Come

Yoga master B.K.S. Iyengar designed this way of practicing Downward- and Upward-Facing Dog Pose, the Supported Headstand hanging in the ropes and other rope movements. At his institute in India and in yoga centers around the world, the lower and upper ropes are attached to hooks in the wall, as illustrated.

For more detailed instructions on using yoga wall ropes, please see the Yoga Props Wall Ropes Usage Guide listed in the Resources section. See also the photographs and instructions in the classic, *Yoga: A Gem for Women,* by Geeta Iyengar. Wall ropes are beneficial for all ages, but I consider them essential for women during the menopause transition and beyond. Especially if you have a desk job and sit long hours behind a computer, they are the antidote for the stiffness that tends to settle into the body during menopause. Yoga wall ropes can be purchased as a kit, complete with all hardware and instructions. For the price of a manicure, pedicure and facial, you can purchase wall ropes and enjoy the health benefits for years to come.

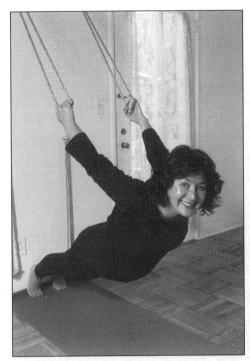 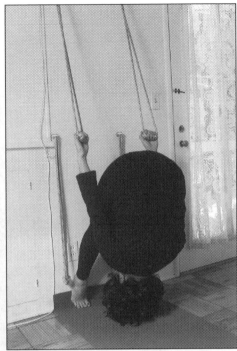

Upward-Facing Dog and Forward Bend with yoga ropes. Yoga ropes stretch and strengthen the whole body and tone pelvic and abdominal organs.

Downward-Facing Dog Pose with Wall Ropes (Adho Mukha Svanasana)

How to practice: I highly recommend purchasing professional yoga wall ropes from your local yoga center or the prop sources listed at the back of this book. You can also make a loop that is approximately six feet long out of soft rope, mountain climbing webbing or other strap. You will need an open door with two sturdy doorknobs and a yoga sticky mat to keep you from slipping. Loop the belt around the doorknobs and step into it, placing it at the crease at the top of your thighs. Lean forward into the rope until your weight feels supported. When you feel secure and the rope is taut, bring your

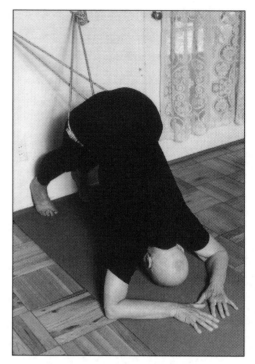

*Hanging in the ropes, arms can be straight,
actively stretching, or relaxed, as illustrated.*

hands to the floor on your mat and walk your feet back
toward the door. Your body should form an upside-down
V shape. Stay in this pose for at least one minute,
breathing softly and allowing the spine to lengthen.

To come out of the pose, walk your hands and feet
toward each other, lean into the belt and inhale as you
come up. This pose is well worth learning under the
guidance of an instructor.

Benefits: Hanging Downward-Facing Dog Pose and
other halfway upside-down poses that place the head
below the level of the heart stimulate the endocrine system, including the pituitary gland, which helps regulate
the changes in hormone levels that occur during

menopause. Hanging from a rope allows you to hold the pose longer, giving the back of the body a delicious stretch. The gentle traction of this pose elongates the spinal column, eases back and neck pain and helps restore an open, youthful posture.

Caution: If the backs of your legs are very stiff or if you have back problems, place your arms on the seat of a chair in front of you.

Supported Headstand Hanging from a Rope or Pelvic Sling (Sirsasana)

My students going through menopause crave hanging upside down. There is no strain on the neck involved in practicing this supported variation of the classic Headstand. It does not require any muscular effort. Women who feel agitated or heated and who do not get good results practicing the classic Headstand during menopause say that the Supported Headstand has a quiet, gently energizing effect.

Benefits: In this Supported Headstand using yoga wall ropes, the pituitary and the adrenal glands as well as the generative organs receive the benefit of improved oxygenation. This gives the mind and body a peaceful and energetic feeling. Remember that in the inverted poses, blood supply to the brain, head and neck is improved with no extra effort on the heart. Better circulation improves functioning not only to the brain but to the endocrine glands located in the head and neck. The feeling of increased energy and revitalization in the body and brain that occurs after practicing inversions cannot be overemphasized during the menopause transition.

Caution: While halfway upside-down poses and

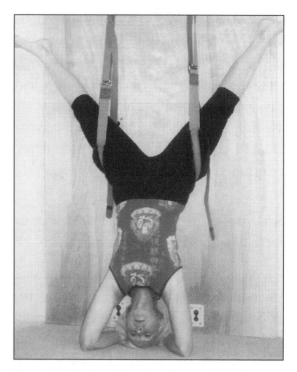

Supported Headstand hanging from a pelvic sling.

gentle inversions like *Viparita Karani* are safe for most people, turning the body completely upside down is not appropriate for everyone, especially if you are a newcomer to yoga. Hanging completely upside down is not recommended during menstruation or for women with hiatal hernias, eye pressure problems, retinal problems, heart problems or anyone using blood thinners. For women new to practicing inversions, it is wise to practice halfway upside-down poses like Downward-Facing Dog Pose (either hanging from the rope or the classic weight-bearing pose practiced with the hands on the floor) before turning your body completely upside down. Increase the length of time you stay in the pose gradually and rest in Child's Pose for at least one minute when you come down.

Since this is an important pose for women during menopause, it is shown here. Inversion slings and other inversion devices generally come with instructions, but it is best to have a knowledgeable teacher present to assist you with proper technique until you are familiar with inverting yourself safely. I recommend that you learn all inverted poses under the guidance of an experienced teacher.

Lying Back Over a Backbender
(*Viparita Dandasana* on a Backbender)

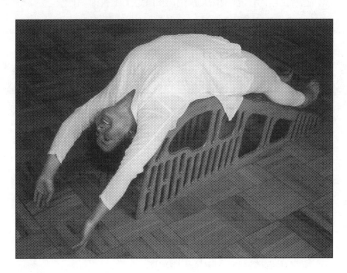

I recommend that if you have to choose between buying a new couch or a backbender that you choose a backbender!

When your muscles are too tight or weak, or you are afraid of putting your body in positions or shapes that it has not been in for many years, props are a way of removing the obstacles between you and a pose that seems out of reach. With the backbender, available for use at many yoga centers or prop companies, almost anyone can begin to practice a safe, supported backbend. The backbender supports and lengthens your spine; stretches your arms and shoulders; opens your rib cage and lungs; deepens your breathing; and stretches the groin, abdomen and front of thighs.

Lying on the backbender opens your chest and counteracts the rounding of the upper back. If you have neck or back problems, learn to use the backbender and more challenging poses, such as Lying Back Over a Chair, with the help of a qualified instructor. Most beginners need extra support under their head, neck or back.

Section VI: Key Poses to Learn Under the Guidance of an Experienced Teacher

- **Lying Back Over a Chair**—Inverted Staff Pose *(Viparita Dandasana* on a chair*)*
- **Supported Shoulderstand with Chair** *(Salamba Sarvangasana)*
- **Supported Half Plow Pose with Chair** *(Ardha Halasana)*
- **Supported Shoulderstand Variation** *(Niralamba Sarvangasana* with a chair*)*

Here are some additional key poses that help balance the endocrine system during menopause. For experienced students, other inversions, such as the classic Headstand *(Sirsasana)* and active backbends requiring strength and exertion, can be beneficial depending on your energy level and your individual response to the pose.

Lying Back Over a Chair—Inverted Staff Pose
(*Viparita Dandasana* on a chair)

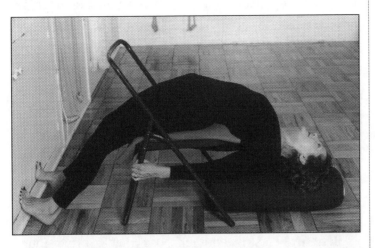

How to practice: Place a sturdy chair (a yoga folding chair is best) about two feet away from a wall. The exact distance depends on your leg length—far enough so that when you straighten your legs you can place your toes or entire foot, as illustrated, on the wall. Place a folded sticky mat or blanket over the front edge of the seat. Sit backward on the chair, facing the wall, with your legs through the chair as illustrated. Scoot your bottom toward the wall in front of you so that when you lean back, your head and neck extend past the chair seat and your shoulder blades drape over the edge of the seat. Hold onto the sides of the chair as you slowly arch backwards.

If you have a long upper body and your shoulder blades drape too far over the chair seat, scoot your bottom farther toward the back edge of the seat (toward the wall in front of you). Take your feet toward the wall, and as you straighten your legs, press your feet into the wall as illustrated. The photo illustrates how you can rest your head on a bolster and blankets and various arm positions to help open your chest. If you are a beginner or if you feel any discomfort in your back, place your feet higher up against the wall as illustrated on page 59, or on a bolster or other height, so that your feet are level with your pelvis. Beginners can stay for about thirty seconds to one minute. Experienced practitioners can increase the length of time gradually and benefit greatly from a long stay in this pose.

To come out, bend your knees, place your feet on the floor close to the chair, hold onto the back of the chair and carefully come up, lifting the chest. It is restful to gently lean forward over the back of the chair. Carefully come out of the chair. Rest in Child's Pose.

Benefit: This is another pose that I often found myself referring to as "menopause medicine" as I went through the change. On mornings when my energy was low, practicing this pose gave me the energy to teach my classes. Supported backbends such as Lying Back Over a Chair have a powerful physiological effect on the nervous system, glands and organs. You can feel the massage of your inner organs during a long stay in this pose. The chest expands, opening the heart center and releasing negativity from the body. You will feel emotionally cleansed after practicing this pose. It removes depression and lifts your spirits.

Caution: I recommend that you learn this pose under the guidance of an experienced teacher. If you have back or neck problems your teacher can show you how to place props to support your head, neck and back in this pose.

Supported Shoulderstand with Chair
(Salamba Sarvangasana)

How to Practice: Place a sturdy chair on a non-slippery surface and place a bolster or two folded blankets directly in front of the chair legs to support your shoulders. Place a folded sticky mat or folded blanket over the front edge seat of the chair. Sitting on the chair, bring your legs over the back. Holding onto the chair, lower your shoulders to the blankets and the back of your head to the floor.

Benefits: This is considered the "queen" or "mother" of all the yoga poses. It is a key pose for balancing the endocrine system, cooling hot flashes and giving the whole body a tune up and "spring cleaning." If you want to quiet your mind and turn off the noise in your head,

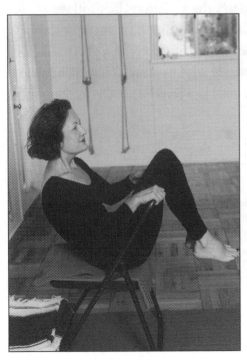
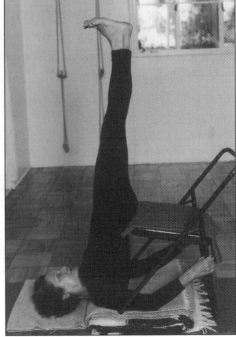

practice Shoulderstand! According to Iyengar, Shoulder-stand alleviates hypertension; relieves breathlessness and heart palpitations; improves the functioning of the thyroid and parathyroid glands; helps relieve insomnia and soothes the nervous system; relieves congestion and heaviness in the ovaries; helps to treat ovarian cysts, prolapsed uterus and reduces uterine fibroids; alleviates urinary disorders and improves elimination. Due to inverting the body, blood flows easily to the organs, especially the liver, the largest organ in the body. It is also a key pose for boosting the immune system and helps treat colds, throat problems and sinus congestion.

Caution: Do not do this pose or any other inverted poses when menstruating. Seek the advice of an experienced teacher if you have back or neck problems, osteoporosis, high blood pressure or heart problems before practicing this pose or the variations that follow.

Note: If you find it too difficult or uncomfortable to practice Supported Shoulderstand with a chair, ask your teacher how to practice with the help of a wall, as shown in the book, *The New Yoga for People Over 50.*

Supported Half Plow Pose with Chair
(Ardha Halasana)

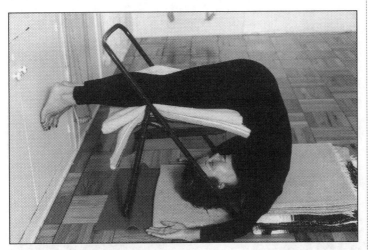

Supported Half Plow Pose with Chair.

How to Practice: This pose follows Supported Shoulderstand or can be practiced on its own. Note in the photo that the legs are supported by the chair seat, allowing your body to relax completely while your organs invert. Depending on your height, place two or three folded blankets on the chair seat so that your spine is extended in the pose. The shoulders are supported by two or three folded blankets as in Shoulderstand, placed near the legs of the chair. Lie with your shoulders on the blankets and your head under the chair seat. Bend your knees to your chest and swing your legs over your head. Move your bottom toward your feet so that your thighs completely rest on the chair seat. Relax your arms back, palms facing up. A teacher can show you how to make this healing pose truly comfortable.

Benefits: Deeply relaxing for the mind and nervous system.

Supported Shoulderstand Variation (Niralamba Sarvangasana with a Chair)

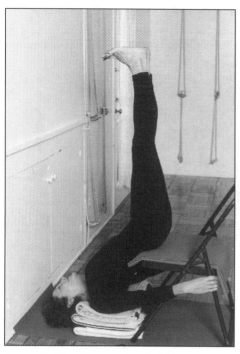

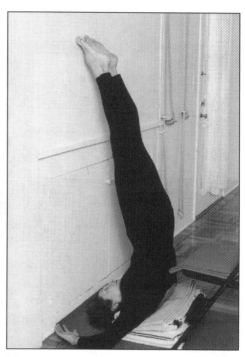

Supported Shoulderstand variation.   **Niralamba Sarvangasana.**

How to Practice: This pose can be learned after you master Supported Shoulderstand. It is best to seek the advice of an instructor trained in this pose.

Benefits: *Light On Yoga,* by B.K.S. Iyengar, gives several pages of benefits for Supported Shoulderstand and this variation, *Niralamba Sarvangasana.* The tremendous effect of this pose on the endocrine and nervous systems during menopause cannot be over emphasized. It is ideal for replenishing your energy reserves at the end of the day. For experienced students, according to Geeta Iyengar, it is even more effective for easing hot flashes than Supported Shoulderstand.

Note: All of these poses can be practiced without the support of a chair. Using support allows you to relax and hold the pose longer, thus increasing the benefits.

As you become familiar with these postures, please remember that a yoga program for women's health problems includes other poses and variations that are best learned under the guidance of a yoga teacher. Your instructor may give you specific, individualized instructions to follow. Be aware that in practicing yoga, there are subtle adjustments and refinements to poses that cannot be covered in a book. I strongly encourage you to seek and work with a knowledgeable teacher who can help you make yoga a supportive companion during menopause and the years beyond.

Ana Forrest, age 46

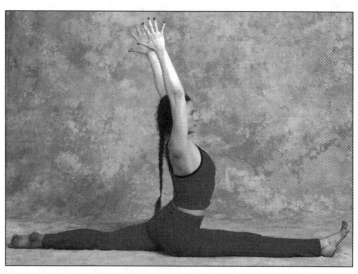

This asana is dedicated to Hanuman, a powerful monkey chief of extraordinary strength and prowess. This pose commemorates his fabulous leaps across the sea to the tops of the Himalayas. Hanumanasana represents a "leap in consciousness" or a movement from one shore to the other or one stage of life to the next.

Strength and Spirit

The way we think about menopause needs to be reframed. We need to understand that the cycles of life are gates of initiation. We can use these changing times to step through the gates, explore our mysteries, shatter the chrysalis and unfold our wings. This can be an exciting time of cultivating and growing our wisdom. You choose: Do you choose fear and diminishing yourself? Or do you choose to explore the mysterious and unknown aspects of yourself?

In yoga, menopause can be a breakthrough time. It involves learning to work authentically and more honestly; tuning into your energy flows and blocks and feeling how they have patterned your neuro-musculature; then applying your breath and your poses to the areas needing help.

Many of the women I work with are delighted to explore new fields of physical, mental and emotional prowess. We can inspire ourselves—one another and our young people—by being a living example of potential actualized. We can model a different, much more enticing future for our young people to look forward to, instead of being ignored and devalued because we're over a certain age. We fully grown women can embody and model the beauty of a rich spirit versus just a wrinkle-free face.

The natural female cycles of menstruation, pregnancy, perimenopause and menopause are treasures of discovery. They contain the elements of our own unique magic. It is during these cycles that we can learn to transform our experiences into healing "medicine" instead of viewing them as poisonous and inconvenient annoyances.

This attitude of respect for women and their growth cycles is what I teach in yoga. You can create ways that develop your connection to the sacred right on your mat. For me, yoga is my daily ceremony of cleansing my mind and cell tissue of the smog of life. A time to delve into the mystery, a time to delight and nourish my soul. I invite you to join me on the mat.

Your yoga practice can provide a private, safe arena in which you listen to your internal signals, the buried and suffocated parts of yourself. As you move more deeply into a yoga pose, you listen to your body. Listen, feel for your first edge of resistance. When your body resists, it is saying, "wait." If you wait and breathe into that tugging place, there can be an opening like an internal flowering that upgrades, in a moment, the quality of energy you have inside. If you just barge on past that signal, occupied with where you think you should be in the pose, you are shunning the voice of your body's intelligence.

Yoga is all about returning over and over again to the present moment—finding out what is happening right now and responding to that. When we activate and direct our curiosity, we begin to discover our potential. Thus begins the healing of our physical, mental, emotional and spiritual bodies. This change in the way we perceive ourselves transforms the way we walk our life road—and ripples that beauty into the world. This is our contribution to healing on a planetary level. Women, let us begin to lay a premise in honoring ourselves. What we have to gain ultimately is our entire life.

To me, what is important is to *wake up!* Wake up and follow the dictates of my spirit.

The Buddha said, "If you want to know what your future will be like, then look at your life right now." Each action we take now forms the cobblestones of our path into the future.

Ana Forrest, founder of the Forrest Yoga Circle, celebrates the beauty of life and the power of spirit in her yoga. Trained in a multitude of healing modalities, including Native American medicine and ritual, she guides her students toward healing by teaching them how to change their relationship to their past and how to discover, nourish and infuse their spirit into all parts of their lives.

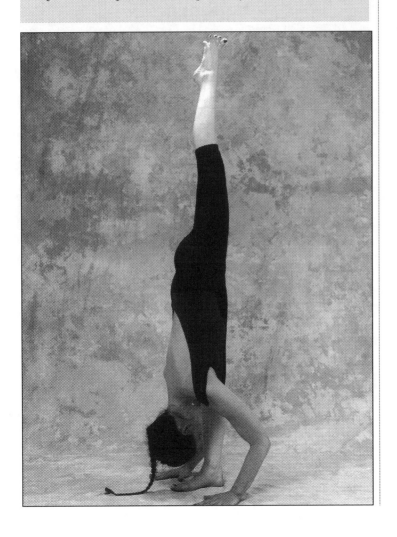

Resources

꒰

Most of the Web sites listed here link to numerous other Web sites that can answer your questions about yoga, and help you find teachers, yoga centers in your area, workshops on yoga and menopause, and sources for yoga books, props and videos.

Yoga with Suza Francina

Suza Francina teaches at Sacred Space, a yoga center located in Ojai, California. For information about Suza's teaching schedule, visit her Web site at *www.suzafrancina.com.* Or contact her at:

Suza Francina
P.O. Box 1258
Ojai, CA 93024
(805) 646-4673
E-mail: *Sfrancina@aol.com*
www.suzafrancina.com

Yoga Teachers Featured in This Book

Gaye Abbott
www.yogahereandnow.com

Ingrid Boulting
www.ingridboulting.com

Linda DiCarlo
www.lindadicarlo.com

Ana Forrest
www.forrestyoga.com

Diana Rose Hartman
E-mail: *Dianahartwoman@aol.com*

Denise Lampron
E-mail: *Deniselampron@aol.com*

243

Judith Lasater   **Dale Mirmow**
www.judithlasater.com   E-mail: *mirmow@earthlink.net*

Julie Lawrence   **Patricia Walden**
www.jlyc.com   *www.Yogawisdom.com*

Virginia Lee   **Susan Winter Ward**
E-mail: *bhakti.2u@juno.com*   *www.yogaheart.com*

Maggie Mellor
www.easeintoyoga.com

Finding a Teacher in Your Area

B.K.S. Iyengar Yoga National Association of the United States, Inc.
(800) 889-YOGA
www.iyaus.org

***Yoga Journal's* Yoga Teachers Directory**
Provides a directory of teachers internationally and articles on
all aspects of yoga.
2054 University Ave, Suite 600
Berkeley, CA 94704
(800) 359-YOGA
www.yogajournal.com

***Yoga International's* Guide to Yoga Teachers and Classes**
RR1, P.O. Box 1130
Honesdale, PA 18431
(570) 253-4929
www.Yimag.org

Yoga Research and Education Center (YREC)
P.O. Box 426
Manton, CA 96059
(530) 474-5700
mail@yrec.org
www.yrec.org

International Association of Yoga Therapists (IAYT)
P.O. Box 426
Manton, CA 96059
(530) 474-5700
mail@iayt.org
www.iayt.org

Yoga Alliance
This professional organization for yoga teachers can refer you to teachers in your area.
122 W. Lancaster Ave., Suite 204
Reading, PA 19607-1874
(877) 964-2255
www.yogalliance.org
info@yogalliance.org

Kripalu Center for Yoga and Health
Offers women's health workshops year-round, including *Natural Medicine and Yoga for Menopause* with Lorilee Schoenbeck, N.D., and *Woman Heal Thyself* with Nischala Joy Devi.
P.O. Box 793
West Street
Lenox, MA 01240-0793
(800) 741-SELF
www.kripalu.org

Yoga and Health Professionals

Wouldn't it be nice if the next time you went in for a checkup there was a back-bender and other yoga props in the waiting room so you could stretch and relax while waiting for the doctor to see you? A growing number of medical and naturo-pathic doctors are using yoga to help treat various health problems. Some specialize in menopause and women's health issues. For information about health professionals using yoga, contact the Yoga Research and Education Society, listed under "Finding a Teacher in Your Area." Or go to *www.yogajournal.com* and look for articles such as "Yoga Under the Microscope" by Kathryn Black.

Krishna Raman, M.D.

If your doctor wants to learn more about yoga, send him or her to Dr. Raman's web site. Here is a doctor who practices what he preaches! Dr. Raman himself demonstrates yoga poses both on his web site and in his book, *A Matter of Health: Integration of Yoga and Western Medicine for Prevention and Cure.* Dr. Raman is trained in both western medicine and yoga. He believes in integrating both sciences and has had wide clinical experience in using yoga as the primary modality of treatment in mainstream medicine. He is currently engaged in integrating the two methods in treating his patients. Dr. Raman is an excellent resource for all health professionals seeking to understand how yoga works. His book is available through Iyengar Yoga Centers and Web sites.

Contact: *www.dr.krishnaraman.com.*

Women's Retreats that Offer Yoga

Inward Bound: Global Adventures in Personal Renewal
Jane Fryer and Jennifer Harvey
(202) 944-YOGA
(800) 760-5099
www.inwardbound.com

Tracks of Vermont Retreats for Women
"Time for Yourself is Time Well Spent"
Mary Castner
(802) 645-1938
E-mail: *tracks@exploreVT.com*
www.exploreVT.com

For other listings of women's yoga retreats, see: *www.yogajournal.com.*

Alternative and Conventional Menopause Resources

Women's Health Resources from Christiane Northrup, M.D.

Dr. Northrup's interactive Web site is among the best places to learn more about the wisdom of menopause. Her monthly newsletter, books and videos are highly recommended.
P.O. Box 199
Yarmouth, ME 04096
www.drnorthrup.com

Farida Sharan School of Natural Medicine

Farida Sharan has beeen a visionary and integrative force in the natural healing world for more than thirty years. Her school for natural medicine offers courses in iridology, naturopathy, herbs and living foods.

P.O. Box 7369
Boulder, CO 80306
(888) 593-6173
E-mail: *snm@purehealth.com*
www.purehealth.com

Susun Weed

Susun Weed has been living the simple life for more than thirty years as a herbalist, goat keeper, homesteader and feminist. In addition to being the author of four highly-acclaimed books on herbs and women's health, Susun lectures worldwide as the voice of the Wise Woman tradition and directs the activities of the Wise Woman Center.

www.susunweed.com
www.ashtreepublishing.com

Miscellaneous Yoga and Menopause Web Sites and Associations

Menopause Literature

For excellent articles about menopause by Arielle Kaph, go to:
www.menstruation.com

Internet: Yoga and Menopause

A general Web search for "Yoga and Menopause" will yield many interesting articles on alternative views about menopause.

The North American Menopause Society

P.O. Box 94527
Cleveland, OH 44101
(440) 422-7550
E-mail: *info@menopause.org*
www.menopause.org

Women's Health Initiative (WHI)

The WHI was established in 1991 by the National Institutes of Health to study the health issues of postmenopausal women. This research program was designed to investigate the causes of heart disease, cancer and osteoporosis. These studies of 167,000 women are examining hormone replacement therapy, nutrition and various promising approaches to disease prevention.

1 Rockledge Center, Suite 300, MS 7966

Bethesda, MD 20892

(301) 402-2900

www.nhlbi.nih.gov/whi

Information About the Source of Premarin

The first limb or moral principle of yoga is *Ahimsa,* which means nonviolence or noninjury. What many women do not realize is that Premarin is composed of estrogenic compounds derived from the urine of pregnant mares (*pre*gnant *mar*e ur*ine*). To obtain estrogen from mares, the horses are artificially inseminated and forced to spend their eleven-month pregnancies in stalls so small they cannot turn. If they try to lie down, their heads are jolted upright by halter chains. Long lines of pregnant horses stand, chained and strapped into cramped concrete and steel pens, like rows of four-legged galley slaves. They shuffle uncomfortably from hoof to hoof. A forlorn look fills their eyes as they stare. Their coats are dull, their ears droopy—telltale signs of a horse's misery. Many get sore, swollen legs or become crippled from standing, months on end, in their tiny concrete stalls.

The mares are kept constantly thirsty. They are denied water so that their urine becomes thick. If they were allowed to drink as much as a normal horse needs, it would overdilute their estrogen. A rubber, medieval-looking "pee bag" and harness is strapped to the mares' vagina by elastic hoses, secured around their flanks and run over a pulley to the ceiling above them, causing sores which are left open and untreated. Most mares develop painful urinary tract infections due to the inhumane conditions.

This treatment is for their entire lives, which only last for the years they are capable of foaling. Once they can no longer become pregnant, the mares will be shot for horsemeat—just like the majority of their unwanted foals—their reward for producing the billions of dollars made from the estrogen drugs prescribed to unaware women.

There are numerous cruelty-free, plant-based and synthetic alternatives to Premarin. Tens of thousands of women have been using these alternatives to treat their menopausal symptoms with success—and with compassion.

For more information contact:

United Animal Nations

United Animal Nations is a nonprofit animal advocacy group with a disaster rescue program, aid for emergency veterinary care and an anti-Premarin campaign.
5892A South Land Park Drive
P.O. Box 188890
Sacramento, CA 95818
(916) 429-2457
Fax: (916) 429-2456
www.uan.org
E-mail: *info@uan.org*
2001-2002 United Animal Nations

Yoga Props

Many yoga Web sites sell yoga props directly or have links to prop companies. You may also be able to purchase props at your local yoga center and other locations. I am familiar with the companies below and their catalogs and Web sites show how to use yoga props.

Bheka Yoga Supplies
258 Ast. #6
Ashland, Oregon 97520
(800) 366-4541
www.Bheka.com

Hugger-Mugger Yoga Products
31 W. Gregson Ave.
Salt Lake City, UT 84115
(800) 473-4888
www.Huggermugger.com

The Great Yoga Wall
(wall rope system)
(775) 781-0468
E-mail: *info@yogawall.com*
www.yogawall.com

Yoga Props
(This company carries wall ropes.)
3055 23rd St.
San Francisco, CA 94110
(888) 856-YOGA
www.yogaprops.net

YogaPro (wall rope system)
(800) 488-6414
www.yogapro.com

Yoga Programs for Heart Disease, Cancer and Other Illnesses

Contact your local yoga center or the Yoga Research and Education Society for programs in your area.

Joanna Colwell

Joanna teaches Iyengar-style yoga and conducts breast-health
workshops around the U.S.
Otter Creek Yoga
P.O. Box 203
Ripton, VT 05766
www.ottercreekyoga.com
E-mail: *joannna@ottercreekyoga.com*

Nischala Joy Devi

Nischala Joy Devi developed the pioneering yoga programs for Drs. Dean Ornish and Michael Lerner. She teaches Yoga of the Heart Training. This is a certification course offered to yoga teachers who want to share therapeutic yoga with people living with heart disease, cancer and other debilitating diseases. It is also useful for people with family histories and/or risk factors for heart disease, cancer and other illnesses.
P.O. Box 346
Fairfax, CA 94978
(415) 459-5336
www.abundantwellbeing.com
E-mail: *Nd@abundantwellbeing.com*

Yoga and Cancer Videos

Gentle Yoga for Breast Cancer Survivors with Esther Myers. Seventy-minute video; $16.00.

Toronto-based teacher Esther Myers, who is a survivor of both the physical and emotional scars of breast cancer, has produced a highly recommend video: *Gentle Yoga for Breast Cancer Survivors.* She has been teaching yoga for nearly twenty-five years. After her mastectomy in 1994, she was invited to develop a yoga program at the Marvelle Koffler Breast Centre, Mt. Sinai Hospital, Toronto, Canada. She is the author of *Yoga and You,* and has produced an audio-guided relaxation tape.

Her video demonstrates a gentle, intelligent, caring practice for all survivors—whether or not they are yoga students—and serves as an essential tool in the self-healing process. This video is based upon what Esther learned from her own struggle with breast cancer and a quarter-century of yoga teaching experience. She understands firsthand the numerous physical benefits yoga practice offers survivors, such as: improved flexibility and mobility; lymph circulation; strength, stability and posture; and decreased stress and fatigue. In addition to the physical trauma of breast cancer and its treatment, Myers also addresses serious emotional issues that can arise, such as anger, grief and self-rejection. In her introduction to the session, and at frequent intervals throughout the session, she conveys a message of positive self-acceptance. This video can be ordered from *www.yogajournal.com*.

Yoga and the Gentle Art of Healing: A Journey of Recovery After Breast Cancer with Susan Rosen. Forty-three-minute video; $19.95.

Susan Rosen, a California yoga teacher, is also a breast cancer survivor. The practice on this highly recommended video focuses not only on the upper-body limitations created by mastectomy and radiation therapy, but also on the mental scars of the treatment. Includes clear instructions on practicing postures and on easing discomfort in yoga poses with the appropriate use of props.

To order the video, contact Susan Rosen at: *www.yogajoyofdelmar.com*.

Susan's video is available at *www.yogajournal.com*.

(858) 481-3912
E-mail: *yogajoy@hotmail.com*

Bibliography

Menopause and Women's Health

Agosta, Carolyn. *Baby Boomers' Menopause Handbook: Through the Other End of Puberty.* Gualala, CA: CA Publishing, Ink, 2000.

Airola, Paavo, Ph.D. N.D. *Everywoman's Book: Practical Guide to Holistic Health.* Phoenix, AZ: Health Plus Publishers, 1979.

Appleton, Nancy, Ph.D. *Lick the Sugar Habit.* Avery, 1996.

Ballentine, Rudolph, M.D. *Diet & Nutrition: A Holistic Approach.* Honesdale, PA: The Himalayan International Institute, 1978.

Bieler, Henry G., M.D. *Food Is Your Best Medicine.* New York: Random House, 1965.

Borysenko, Joan, Ph.D. *A Woman's Book of Life: The Biology, Psychology, and Spirituality of the Feminine Life Cycle.* New York: Penguin Putnam, Inc., 1996.

Brennan, Barbara Ann. *Hands of Light: A Guide to Healing Through the Human Energy Field.* New York: Bantam Doubleday Dell Publishing Group, Inc., 1988.

Brown, Susan E., Ph.D. and Russell Jaffe, M.D. *Better Bones, Better Body: Beyond Estrogen and Calcium.* Contemporary Books, 2000. [Contact: (315) 432-0231; *www.betterbones.com*].

Budoff, Penny Wise, M.D. *No More Hot Flashes—And Other Good News.* New York: Warner Books, 1983.

Diamond, John W., M.D., W. Lee Cowden, M.D., and Burton Goldberg. *An Alternative Medicine Definitive Guide to Cancer.* Tiburon, CA: Future Medicine Publishing, Inc., 1997.

Dosh, Robert M., Ph.D., Susan N. Fukushima, M.D., Jane E. Lewis, Ph.D., Robert L. Ross, M.D., and Lynne A. Steinman, Ph.D. *The Taking Charge of Menopause Workbook.* Oakland, CA: New Harbinger Publications, Inc., 1997.

Evans, William, Ph.D. Irwin H. Rosenberg, M.D., and Jacqueline Thompson, *Biomarkers: The 10 Keys to Prolonging Vitality.* New York: Simon & Schuster, Inc., 1991.

Frahm, Dave. *A Cancer Battle Plan Sourcebook: A Step-by-Step Health Program to Give Your Body a Fighting Chance.* New York: Tarcher/Putnam, 2000.

Gaby, Alan, M.D. *Preventing & Reversing Osteoporosis,* Prima Publishing, 1994.

Gerber, Richard, M.D. *Vibrational Medicine: The #1 Handbook of Subtle-Energy Therapies.* Rochester, VT: Bear & Co., 2001.

Hoffman, Lisa and Alison Freeland. *The Healing Power of Movement: How to Benefit from Physical Activity During Your Cancer Treatment.* Cambridge, MA: Perseus Publishing, 2002.

Khalsa, Gurucharan Singh, Ph.D. and Yogi Bhajan, Ph.D. *Breathwalk: Breathing Your Way to a Revitalized Body, Mind, and Spirit.* New York: Random House/Broadway Books, 2000.

Kortge, Carolyn Scott. *The Spirited Walker: Fitness Walking for Clarity, Balance and Spiritual Connection.* San Francisco, CA: Harper Collins, 1998.

Krucoff, Carol and Mitchell Krucoff, M.D. *Healing Moves: How to Cure, Relieve, and Prevent Common Ailments with Exercise.* New York: Crown Publishing, 2000.

Lark, Susan, M.D. *Premenstrual Syndrome Self-Help Book: A Woman's Guide to Feeling Good All Month.* Los Angeles: Forman Publishing, Inc., 1984.

——————. *The Menopause Self-Help Book: A Woman's Guide to Feeling Wonderful for the Second Half of Her Life.* Berkeley, CA: Celestial Arts, 1990.

Lee, John R., M.D. *What Your Doctor May Not Tell You About Menopause.* New York: Warner Hopkins, Virginia Books, Inc., 1996.

Lerner, Michael. *Choices in Healing: Integrating the Best of Conventional and Complementary Approaches to Cancer.* Cambridge, MA: The MIT Press, 1994.

Liberman, Jacob, O.D., Ph.D. *Light: Medicine of the Future—How We Can Use It to Heal Ourselves Now.* Santa Fe, NM: Bear & Company, 1991.

Love, Susan M., M.D. *Dr. Susan Love's Hormone Book: Making Informed Choices About Menopause.* New York: Random House, 1997.

Meinig, George, D.D.S. *"New" trition.* Ojai, CA: Bion Publishing, 1987.

Mendelsohn, Robert S., M.D. *Male Practice: How Doctors Manipulate Women.* Chicago, IL: Contemporary Books, Inc., 1981.

Myss, Caroline, Ph.D. *Anatomy of the Spirit: The Seven Stages of Power and Healing.* New York: Crown Publishers, Inc., 1996.

Nelson, Miriam E., Ph.D. and Sarah Wernick, Ph.D. *Strong Women, Strong Bones.* New York: Penguin Putnam Inc., 2000.

Northrup, Christiane, M.D. *The Wisdom of Menopause: Creating Physical and Emotional Health and Healing During the Change.* New York: Random House/Bantam Books, 2001.

——————. *Women's Bodies, Women's Wisdom: Creating Physical and Emotional Health and Healing.* New York: Random House/Bantam Books, 1994.

Ojeda, Linda, Ph.D. *Menopause Without Medicine.* Claremont, CA: Hunter House, Inc., 1989.

Olsen, Andrea and Caryn McHose. *Body Stories: A Guide to Experiential Anatomy.* New York: Station Hill Press, Inc., 1991.

Ornish, Dean, M.D. *Dr. Dean Ornish's Program For Reversing Heart Disease.* New York: Random House, 1990.

Oz, Memet, M.D. *Healing from the Heart: A Leading Surgeon Combines Eastern and Western Traditions to Create the Medicine of the Future.* East Rutherford, NJ: Plume Books, 1999.

Padus, Emrika. *The Woman's Encyclopedia of Health & Natural Healing.* Emmaus, PA: Rodale Press, 1981.

Pert, Candace B., Ph.D. *Molecules of Emotion: Why You Feel the Way You Feel.* New York: Scribner, 1997.

Price, Weston A., D.D.S. *Nutrition and Physical Degeneration.* New York: Harper & Brothers, 1939.

Schwarzbein, Diana, M.D., Deville, Nancy. *The Schwarzbein Principle: The Truth About Losing Weight, Being Healthy and Feeling Younger.* Deerfield, FL: Health Communications, Inc., 1999.

Schoenbeck, Lorilee, N.D., Gibson, Cheryl A., M.D. and Barss, M. Brooke, M.D. *Menopause: Bridging the Gap Between Natural and Conventional Medicine.* New York: Kensington Publishing Corp., 2002.

Sellman, Sherrill. *Hormone Heresy: What Women Must Know About Their Hormones.* Victoria, Australia: Get Well International, 1998.

Sharan, Farida, N.D., M.H. *Creative Menopause: Illuminating Women's Health & Spirituality.* Colorado: Wisdom Press, 1994.

Sheehy, Gail. *The Silent Passage: Menopause.* New York: Random House, 1991.

Smith, Kathy. *Moving Through Menopause: The Complete Program for Exercise, Nutrition, and Total Wellness.* New York: AOL Time Warner, 2002.

Spilner, Maggie. *Prevention's Complete Book of Walking: Everything You Need to Know to Walk Your Way to Better Health.* Emmaus, PA: Rodale, Inc., 2000.

Tiwari, Bri. Maya. *The Path of Practice: A Woman's Book of Ayurvedic Healing.* New York: Random House/Ballantine Books, 2000.

Weed, Susun S. *Menopausal Years: The Wise Woman Way.* Woodstock, NY: Ash Tree Publishing, 1992.

——————. *Breast Cancer? Breast Health!: The Wise Woman Way.* Woodstock, NY: Ash Tree Publishing, 1996.

——————. *New Menopausal Years: The Wise Woman Way.* Woodstock, NY: Ash Tree Publishing, 2002.

Weiss, Kay, ed. *Women's Health Care: A Guide to Alternatives.* Reston, VA: Prentice-Hall, 1984.

Wise, Sabina J. *The Sugar Addict's Diet.* East Canaan, CT: New Century Publishing, 2000.

Women's Spirituality and Psychology

Allione, Tsultrim. *Women of Wisdom.* London, UK: Routledge & Kegan Paul Ltd., 1984.

Anderson, Sherry Ruth and Patricia Hopkins. *The Feminine Face of God: The Unfolding of The Sacred In Women.* New York: Bantam Books, 1991.

Angier, Natalie. *Woman: An Intimate Geography.* New York: Random House, 2000.

Bolen, Jean Shinoda, M.D. *Crossing to Avalon: A Woman's Midlife Pilgrimage.* San Francisco: Harper Collins, 1994.

Cameron, Anne. *Daughters of Copper Woman.* Vancouver, BC: Press Gang Publishers, 1981.

Chernin, Kim. *The Obsession: Reflections on the Tyranny of Slenderness.* New York: Harper & Row, 1981.

Chesler, Phyllis. *Women & Madness.* New York: Doubleday/Avon, 1972.

Chodron, Pema. *When Things Fall Apart: Heart Advice for Difficult Times.* Boston, MA: Shambhala, 2000.

Clow, Barbara Hand. *Liquid Light of Sex: Understanding Your Key Life Passages.* Santa Fe, NM: Bear & Company, 1991.

Conway, Timothy, Ph.D. *Women of Power and Grace: Nine Astonishing, Inspiring Luminaries of Our Time.* Santa Barbara, CA: The Wake Up Press, 1994.

Dalai Lama, H. H. and Howard C. Cutler, M.D. *The Art of Happiness: A Handbook for Living*. New York: Penguin Putnam, 1998.

Dalai Lama, H. H. *Ethics for The New Millenium*. New York: Penguin Putnam, 1999.

Diamant, Anita. *The Red Tent*. New York: Pan Books/Picador, 1997.

Duerk, Judith. *Circle of Stones: Woman's Journey to Herself*. San Diego, CA: LuraMedia, 1989.

Estes, Clarissa Pinkola, Ph.D. *Women Who Run with the Wolves: Myths and Stories of the Wild Woman Archetype*. New York: Ballantine, 1992.

Griffin, Susan. *Woman and Nature: The Roaring Inside Her*. New York: Harper & Row, 1978.

Halifax, Joan. *The Fruitful Darkness: Reconnecting with the Body of the Earth*. San Francisco, CA: Harper Collins, 1993.

Harding, Esther M. *The Way of All Women*. Boston, MA: Shambhala, 1990.

Hayden, Tom. *The Lost Gospel of the Earth: A Call for Renewing Nature, Spirit, & Politics*. San Francisco, CA: The Sierra Club, 1996.

Heilbrun, Carolyn G. *Writing a Woman's Life*. New York: W.W. Norton & Company, 1988.

Hollis, James. *The Middle Passage: From Misery to Meaning in Midlife*. Toronto, Canada: Inner City Books, 1993.

Johnson, Robert A. *Lying with the Heavenly Woman: Understanding and Integrating the Feminine Archetypes in Men's Lives*. San Francisco: Harper Collins, 1994.

Khema, Ayya. *Who Is My Self?: A Guide to Buddhist Meditation*. Somerville, MA: Wisdom Publications, 1997.

——————. *I Give You My Life: The Autobiography of a Western Buddhist Nun*. Somerville, MA: Wisdom Publications, 1997.

Lerner, Harriet G., Ph.D. *The Dance of Deception: Pretending and Truth-Telling in Women's Lives*. New York: Harper Collins, 1993.

Matthews, Caitlin. *Sophia: Goddess of Wisdom, Bride of God*. Wheaton, IL: Quest Books, 2001.

McLaughlin, Corinne and Gordon Davidson. *Spiritual Politics: Changing the World From the Inside Out*. New York: Random House/Ballantine, 1994.

Moran, Victoria. *Lit from Within*. San Francisco, CA: Harper, 2001.

Moseley, Douglas and Naomi Moseley. *The Shadow Side of Intimate Relationships: What's Going on Behind the Scenes*. East Sandwich, MA: North Star Publications, 2000.

Noble, Vicki. *Shakti Woman: Feeling Our Fire, Healing Our World—The New Female Shamanism.* New York: Harper Collins, 1991.

O'Brien, Paddy. *Becoming Yourself.* London, UK: Azure, 2002.

Qualls-Corbett, Nancy. *The Sacred Prostitute: Eternal Aspect of the Feminine.* Toronto, Canada: Inner City Books, 1988.

Resnick, Stella, Ph.D. *The Pleasure Zone: Why We Resist Good Feelings and How to Let Go and Be Happy.* Berkeley, CA: Conari Press, 1997.

Roundtree, Cathleen, ed. *On Women Turning 50: Celebrating Mid-Life Discoveries.* San Francisco, CA: Harper Collins, 1993.

Sakya, Jamyang and Julie Emery. *Princess in the Land of Snows: The Life of Jamyang Sakya in Tibet.* Boston, MA: Shambhala, 1990.

Scott, Mary Hugh. *The Passion of Being Woman: A Love Story From the Past for the Twenty-First Century.* Aspen, CO: MacMurray & Beck Communications, 1991.

Sheehy, Gail. *Pathfinders: Overcoming the Crises of Adult Life and Finding Your Own Path to Well-Being.* New York: Bantam Books, 1981.

————. *New Passages: Mapping Your Life Across Time.* New York: Random House/ Ballantine, 1995.

Starhawk. *The Fifth Sacred Thing.* New York: Bantam Books, 1993.

Steinem, Gloria. *Revolution From Within: A Book of Self-Esteem.* Boston, MA: Little Brown & Company, 1992.

Ueland, Brenda. *If You Want To Write: A Book about Art, Independence and Spirit.* St. Paul, MN: Graywolf Press, 1987.

Walker, Barbara G. *The Crone: Woman of Age, Wisdom, and Power.* San Francisco, CA: Harper Collins, 1985.

————. *The Woman's Encyclopedia of Myths and Secrets.* San Francisco, CA: Harper Collins, 1983.

Waring, Cynthia. *Bodies Unbound: Transforming Lives Through Touch.* Boulder, CO: Books Beyond Borders, 1996.

Williamson, Marianne. *A Woman's Worth.* New York: Random House/Ballantine, 1993.

Wolf, Naomi. *The Beauty Myth: How Images of Beauty Are Used Against Women.* New York: Doubleday-Anchor, 1992.

Wood, Beatrice. *I Shock Myself: The Autobiography of Beatrice Wood.* Ojai, CA: Dillingham Press, 1985.

Zweig, Connie, ed. *To Be a Woman: The Birth of the Conscious Feminine.* New York: Tarcher/Putnam, 1990.

Yoga

Benedick, Linda and Veronica Wirth. *Yoga for Equestrians: A New Path for Achieving Union with the Horse.* North Pomfret, VT: Trafalgar Square Publishing, 2000.

Birch, Beryl Bender. *Power Yoga: The Total Strength and Flexibility Workout.* New York: Simon & Schuster, 1995.

Carrico, Mara. *Yoga Journal's Yoga Basics: The Essential Beginner's Guide to Yoga for a Lifetime of Health and Fitness.* New York: Henry Holt & Co, Inc., 1997.

Cope, Stephen. *Yoga and the Quest for the True Self.* New York: Bantam Books, 1999.

Derrick, Jeanne-Marie. *Yoga for Menstruation: Illustrated Practice Sequences from the Teachings of Iyengar Yoga.* New York: self-published, 2001.

Devi, Nischala Joy. *The Healing Path of Yoga: Time-Honored Wisdom and Scientifically Proven Methods That Alleviate Stress, Open Your Heart, and Enrich Your Life.* New York: Three River Press 2000.

Desikachar, T. K. V. *The Heart of Yoga: Developing A Personal Practice.* Rochester, VT: Inner Traditions International, 1995.

Dworkis, Sam. *Extensions: The 20-Minute-a-Day, Yoga-Based Program to Relax, Release & Rejuvenate the Average Stressed-Out Over-35-Year-Old Body.* New York: Poseidon Press, 1994.

Farhi, Donna. *Yoga Mind, Body & Spirit: A Return to Wholeness for Students of All Levels and Traditions.* New York: Henry Holt, 2000.

Feuerstein, Georg, Ph.D. and Payne, Larry Ph.D. *Yoga for Dummies,* IDG Books, 1999.

Francina, Suza. *The New Yoga for People Over 50: A Comprehensive Guide for Midlife and Older Beginners.* Deerfield, FL: Health Communications, Inc., 1997.

Hamilton, Mina. *Serenity to Go: Calming Techniques for Your Hectic Life.* Oakland, CA: New Harbinger Publications, 2001.

Holleman, Dona. *Centering Down.* Firenze, Italy: Tipografia Giuntina, 1981.

Holleman, Dona and O. Sen-Gupta. *Dancing the Body of Light: The Future of Yoga.* The Netherlands: Pegasus Enterprises, 1999.

Iyengar, Geeta S. *Yoga: A Gem for Women.* Spokane, WA: Timeless Books, 1990.

Lain, Ruth. *Yoga With Y'all South Texas Style.* Corpus Christi, TX: Ruth Lain, 2001.

Lasater, Judith Ph.D., P.T. *Living Your Yoga: Finding the Spiritual in Everyday Life.* Berkeley, CA: Rodmell Press, 2000.

——————. *Relax and Renew: Restful Yoga for Stressful Times.* Berkeley, CA: Rodmell Press, 1995.

Lee, Michael. *Phoenix Rising Yoga Therapy: A Bridge from Body to Soul.* Deerfield, FL: Health Communications, Inc., 1997.

Maddern, Jan. *Yoga Builds Bones: Easy Gentle Stretches That Prevent Osteoporosis.* Boston, MA: Element Books, 2000.

Meeks, Sara. *Safe Yoga for Osteoporosis.* (to be published). Sara also teaches workshops on yoga for osteoporosis at Kripalu Center for Health and other locations. Sara's web site is www.sarameekspt.com.

Mehta, Mira. *How to Use Yoga.* Berkeley, CA: Rodmell Press, 1998.

Mehta, Silvia and Mira and Shyam Mehta. *Yoga the Iyengar Way: The New Definitive Illustrated Guide.* New York: Alfred Knopf, 1990.

Miller, Elise Browning and Carol Blackman. *Life Is a Stretch: Easy Yoga, Anytime, Anywhere.* St. Paul, MN: Llewellyn Publications, 2001.

Myers, Esther. *Yoga & You: Energizing and Relaxing Yoga for New and Experienced Students.* Toronto: Random House of Canada, 1996.

O'Brien, Paddy. *Yoga for Women: Complete Mind and Body Fitness.* San Francisco: Harper Collins, 1991.

Payne, Larry, Ph.D., Richard Usatine, M.D. *Yoga Rx: A Step-by Step Program to Promote Health, Wellness, and Healing for Common Ailments.* New York: Broadway Books, 2002.

Raman, Krishna, M.D. *A Matter of Health: Integration of Yoga & Western Medicine for Prevention & Cure.* Madras, India: Eastwest Books Pvt. Ltd., 1998.

Saraswati, Muktananda Swami. *Nawa Yogini Tantra.* Bihar School of Yoga, Monghyr, India, 1977.

Scaravelli, Vanda. *Awakening the Spine: The Stress-Free New Yoga That Works with the Body to Restore Health, Vitality and Energy.* San Francisco, CA: Harper Collins, 1991.

Schatz, Mary Pullig, M.D. *Back Care Basics: A Doctor's Gentle Yoga Program for Back and Neck Pain Relief.* Berkeley, CA: Rodmell Press, 1992.

Schiffmann, Erich. *Yoga: The Spirit and Practice of Moving into Stillness.* New York: Simon & Schuster, 1996.

Self, Philip. *Yogi Bare: Naked Truth from America's Leading Yoga Teachers.* Nashville, TN:

Cypress Moon Press, 1998.

Sivananda, Radha Swami. *Hatha Yoga: The Hidden Language—Symbols, Secrets, and Metaphor.* Spokane, WA: Timeless Books, 1995.

Sparrowe, Linda, and Patricia Walden. *The Woman's Book of Yoga and Health: A Lifelong Guide to Wellness.* Boston, MA: Shambhala, 2002.

Stewart, Mary. *Yoga Over 50: The Way to Vitality, Health and Energy in the Prime of Life.* London, UK: Little, Brown and Company, 1995.

Taylor, Louise. *The Woman's Book of Yoga: A Journal for Body and Mind.* Boston, MA: Tuttle Publishing, 2001.

Ward, Susan Winter. *Yoga for the Young at Heart: Gentle Stretching Exercises for Seniors.* Santa Barbara, CA: Capra Press, 1994.

Yogananda, Paramahansa. *Autobiography of a Yogi.* Los Angeles, CA: Self-Realization Fellowship, 1946.

Other Books of Interest

Blackman, Sushila. *Graceful Exits: How Great Beings Die.* Trumbull, CT: Weatherhill, Inc., 1997.

Goldberg, Natalie. *Writing Down the Bones: Freeing the Writer Within.* Boston, MA: Shambhala, 1986.

——————. *Wild Mind: Living the Writer's Life.* New York: Bantam, 1990.

Hopcke, Robert H. *There Are No Accidents: Synchronicity and the Stories of Our Lives.* New York: Penguin Putnam, 1997.

Hughes-Calero, Heather. *Writing As a Tool for Self-Discovery.* Carmel, CA: Coastline Publishing, 1988.

Krishnamurti, J. *On Nature and the Environment.* San Francisco, CA: Harper Collins, 1991.

Metzger, Deena. *Writing for Your Life: A Guide and Companion to the Inner Worlds.* San Francisco, CA: Harper Collins, 1992.

Books and Publications By and About B.K.S. Iyengar

The Art of Yoga. London: Unwin Paperbacks, 1985.

Body the Shrine, Yoga Thy Light. Bombay, India: published by B. I. Taraporewala for Iyengar's 60th birthday, 1978 (chapter on Yoga for Women by Geeta Iyengar).

Iyengar: His Life and Work. Palo Alto, CA: Timeless Books, 1987.

Yoga: The Path to Holistic Health. London, UK: Dorling Kindersley Ltd., 2001.

Light on Pranayama. New York: Crossroad, 1981.

Light on Yoga. New York: Schocken, 1979.

Light on the Yoga Sutras of Patanjali. London: Harper Collins, 1993.

70 Glorious Years of Yogachrya B. K. S. Iyengar. Bombay, India: Light on Yoga Research Trust, 1990.

Tree of Yoga. Boston: Shambhala, 1989.

Effect of Asanas and Pranayama on the Endocrine System (Dr. Karandikar); Symposium: Women's Problems, with Geeta Iyengar; Yoga and Medical Science: Yoga for Overall Health (Iyengar).

Therapeutic Yoga Sequences. A collection of therapeutic yoga sequences that were given by the Iyengars to individual students. The particulars regarding each individual student, such as constitution, previous yoga experience and ability, weight, age, and ability to grasp instruction were all factored into that individual's personal prescriptive sequence. Compiled by Lois Steinberg, Ph.D.

Iyengar International Women's Intensive Course Notes. Geeta Iyengar and B.K.S. Iyengar. Produced by Lois Steinberg, Ph.D.

IYNAUS Newsletter, Summer 1993: volume 1, number 1. *Yoga and Women.* Geeta Iyengar.

IYNAUS Newsletter, Winter 1996: vol. 3, no. 1. *Matru Devo Bhava* ("Mother is the Goddess") Geeta Iyengar.

IYNAUS Newsletter, Winter 1996: vol. 3, no. 1. *Supported Niralamba Sarvangasana for Humankind.* Lois Steinberg, Ph.D.

IYNAUS Newsletter, Spring 2002: vol. 6, no. 1. *Yoga Research and Therapy: An Overview.* Lois Steinberg, Ph.D.

Iyengar Yoga Odyssey 2001. *Questions & Answers with Geeta Iyengar.* Excerpts from IYASC Q&A Session, Los Angeles, May 8, 2001.

Iyengar Yoga Institute Review

Barnet, Lauren. "The Effects of Yoga on the Circulatory System." (Spring 1999).

Bennett, Susan. "The Effects of Yoga on the Nervous System." (Spring 1999).

Cavanaugh, Carol. "An Interview with Dr. S. V. Karandikar." (February 1984).

Flanigan, Lucy. "The Effects of Yoga on the Respiratory System." (Spring 1999).

Green, Felicity. "Menopause and Yoga." (Fall 1997).

Hondrogen, Dina. "The Effects of Yoga on the Digestive System." (Spring 1999).

Layton, Pat. "Yoga and the Menstrual Cycle." (Fall 1997).

MacLeod, Janet. "Memorable Musings From the Women's Intensive." (Fall 1997).

Moon, Stella. "The Effects of Yoga on the Endocrine System." (Spring 1999).

Transcription of the video on "Menopause" produced by the Institute in Pune, India. Transcript by Kay Parry, with help from Janet Dalmasso and Susan Robertson. Edited by Geeta Iyengar. (January 1996).

Other Periodicals and Publications

Allen, Katie. "Yoga Poses for Women in Breast Cancer Treatment." *Yoga Journal* (Nov/Dec 1998).

Barret, Jenifer. "Heart to Heart." *Yoga Journal* (Nov/Dec 2003).

Black, Kathryn. "Yoga under the Microscope." *Yoga Journal* (Source 2001).

Boucher, Sandy. "Yoga for Cancer. *Yoga Journal"* (May/June 1999).

Cavanaugh, Carol. "Viparita Karani: Supported Inverted Pose." *Yoga Journal* (November/December 1983).

Coldwell, Joanna. "Re-Examining Breast Health." *Yoga Journal* (September/October 2001).

Cole, Roger, Ph.D., "Ask Our Expert: What poses would you recommend to treat adrenal exhaustion?" *www.yogajournal.com.*

Crawford, Amanda McQuade. "Hormones Demystified." *Yoga Journal* (May/June 1997).

Feuerstein, Georg, Ph.D. "Editorial: Whither Yoga Therapy?" *International Journal of Yoga Therapy,* No. 9 (1999).

—————. "Yoga Therapy: Further Ruminations." *International Journal of Yoga Therapy,* No. 11 (2001).

Gudmestad, Julie. "Break Out of Your Slump." *Yoga Journal* (December 2001).

—————. "Face Your Fears of Falling." *Yoga Journal* (July/August 2001).

Kelly, Alice Lesch. "Rest for the Weary." *Yoga Journal* (March/April 2001).

Kraftsow, Gary. "On Yoga Therapy." *Yoga International* (April/May 2002).

Lipson, Elaine. "Yoga Works!" *Yoga Journal* (Winter 1999).

MacMullen, Jane. "Yoga and the Menstrual Cycle." *Yoga Journal* (January/February 1990).

Myers, Esther. "Journey Through Breast Cancer." *Yoga Journal* (November/December 1998).

Ruiz, Fernando Pages. "The Feminine Critique: Most ancient scriptures were written for and by men. Nischala Joy Devi and Esther Myers question their relevance for modern women." *Yoga Journal* (August 2000).

Sander, Ellen. "Moving Through Menopause With Yoga." *Yoga Journal* (February 1996).

Schatz, Mary, M.D. "Yoga Relief for Arthritis: A Pathologist and Yoga Teacher Offers Comprehensive Guidelines for Restoring and Maintaining Joint Health" *Yoga Journal* (May/June 1985); "Yoga, Circulation and Imagery" *Yoga Journal* (January/February 1987); "Restorative Asanas for a Healthy Immune System" *Yoga Journal* (July/August 1987); "You Can Have Healthy Bones! Preventing Osteoporosis with Exercise, Diet and Yoga" *Yoga Journal* (March/April 1988); "Exercises and Yoga Poses for Those at Risk for Osteoporotic Fractures" *Yoga Journal* (March/April 1988); "Yoga and Aging" *Yoga Journal* (May/June 1990); "Relief for Your Aching Back" *Yoga Journal* (May/June 1992).

Stark, John. "Change Your Posture, Change Your Mood." *Yoga Journal* (August 2002).

Walden, Patricia. "Asanas to Relieve Depression." *Yoga Journal* (November/December 1999).

Weintraub, Amy. "The Natural Prozac." *Yoga Journal* (November/December 1999).

——————. "Depression and Our Forgotten Magnificence." *Yoga International* (July/August 2002).

Yoshikawa, Yoko. "Everybody Upside-Down." *Yoga Journal* (September/October 2000).

——————. "Inversions and Menstruation." *Yoga Journal* (September/October 2000).

Willoughby, Deborah. "Radical Wholeness: A Conversation with Rudolph Ballentine, M.D." *Yoga International* (February/March 2000).

Miscellaneous Publications

Abbot, Gaye, C.M.T., I.Y.T. "Yoga and Osteoporosis." *Share Guide* (Jan/Feb 2000).

Dunn, Mary. "In Praise of Props: Utilizing the Mundane to Effect the Miraculous." Yoga '87 Conference Publication.

Eskenazi, Kay and Ruth Steiger. "Backbending Bench Usage Guide," "Eyebag Usage Guide," "Halasana Bench Usage Guide," "Headstander Usage Guide," "Pelvic Swing Usage Guide," "Pranayama Bolster Usage Guide," "Wall Ropes Usage Guide." These booklets are highly recommended and may be purchased through Yoga Props.

Randolph, Bonnie. "Return to Life: How I Defied My Doctor and Survived Ovarian Cancer." *East West Journal* (November/December 1991).

Taylor, Matthew. Article on Yoga and Osteoporosis. Available online at *www.yogatherapy.com.*

Paulhus, Marc. "A Bitter Pill." *California Sun* (Fall 2001).

Stoehn, Bonnie. "The Suffering Behind Premarin: Hurting Horses to Heal Hot Flashes." *Whole Life Times* (May 1994).University of California.

——————. "New Advice About Bone-density Tests." *The University of California, Berkeley Wellness Letter,* (July 2002).

——————. "Hormone Therapy: The Answers Are In." *The University of California, Berkeley Wellness Letter,* (October 2002).

Index of Poses

_ॐ_

Deep Relaxation Pose (*Savasana*) practiced with bolster under legs,
sandbag across abdomen, eyebag over eyes, legs straight, or soles
of the feet together on top of bolster 200
Downward-Facing Dog Pose with Wall Ropes—"Hanging Dog Pose"
(*Adho Mukha Svanasana*) 226
Forward Bend with Wall Ropes 225
Lying Back Over a Backbender (*Viparita Dandasana* on a Backbender) 229
Lying Back Over a Chair-Inverted Staff Pose (*Viparita Dandasana* on a chair) 231
Lying Down Bent Knee Twist Gentle Floor Twist (*Jathara Parivartanasana*). 222
Lying Down (Supine) Big Toe Pose with Leg Opened Up
to Side (*Supta Padangusthasana II*). 219
Seated Bound Angle Pose (*Baddha Konasana*). 217
Seated Wide Angle Pose (*Upavistha Konasana*). 217
Standing Forward Bend with Head Supported on Chair (*Uttanasana*) 204
Supported Bridge Pose—The Menopausal Bridge Pose (*Setu Bandha Sarvangasana*) . 192
Supported Child's Pose (*Adho Mukha Virasana*) 191
Supported Deep Relaxation Pose—The pause that refreshes during
"the pause" (Supported *Savasana*). 186
Supported Downward-Facing Dog Pose (*Adho Mukha Svanasana*) 205
Supported Extended Side Angle Pose (*Utthita Parsvakonasana*) 211
Supported Half Moon Pose (*Ardha Chandrasana*) Back on the Wall 213
Supported Half Moon Pose (*Ardha Chandrasana*) Facing the Wall. 214
Supported Half Plow Pose with Chair (*Ardha Halasana*) 235
Supported Headstand (*Sirsasana*) with Wall Ropes and wide yoga belt
or Inversion Sling 228
Supported Legs Up the Wall Pose—The Great Rejuvenator (*Viparita Karani*) 195
Supported Lying Down Bound Angle Pose—The Goddess Pose
(*Supta Baddha Konasana*). 188
Supported Shoulderstand with Chair (*Salamba Sarvangasana*). 233

Supported Triangle Pose (*Utthita Trikonasana*) 208
Supported Shoulderstand Variation (*Niralamba Sarvangasana*) 236
Supported Warrior II (*Virabhadrasana II*). 210
Upward-Facing Dog Pose with Wall Ropes 225
Wide Angle Standing Forward Bend with Head Supported on Chair
    (*Prasaritta Padotanasana*). 201
Wide Angle Standing Forward Bend with Spine Concave. 202

About the Author

S uza Francina, R.Y.T., is the author of *The New Yoga for People Over 50, A Comprehensive Guide for Midlife and Older Beginners.* She is a certified Iyengar Yoga Instructor and Registered Yoga Teacher with thirty years experience in the field of yoga and exercise therapy. She has written for many publications, including *Yoga Journal,* and is a contributor to *Women's Health Care, A Guide to Alternatives, The Holistic Health Handbook, American Yoga* and *Living Your Yoga.* Her interest in yoga and women's health is related to a wider interest in spiritual politics and the health of the planet. She is a spokesperson for sustainable lifestyles and served as Mayor of Ojai, California, one of the most beautiful and sacred places on Earth. Born in 1949 of Dutch-Indonesian heritage in The Hague, Holland, Suza Francina is the mother of a grown son and daughter and lives with a family that includes several dogs and cats as well as a wise elder potbellied pig.

Healthy Living

Never Be Sick Again

One Disease • Two Causes • Six Pathways

Health Is a Choice Learn How to Choose It

Raymond Francis, M.Sc.
with Kester Cotton

Foreword by
Harvey Diamond
Coauthor of the
#1 *New York Times*
Bestseller *Fit for Life*

Through provocative case studies and cutting-edge scientific research, you will learn an entirely new way to look at health and disease.

Code #9543 • Paperback • $12.95

Containing practical advice, easy-to-follow tips, reference sources and Web sites, this is the one book on health every family needs.

"I recommend this book to all people who want to know how to navigate the confusing world of medicine. Whether you intend to use alternative therapies or to integrate them with conventional medicine, the information in Own Your Health will guide you to making the right decisions."
—**Andrew Weil, M.D.**, author, 8 Weeks to Optimum Health

Own Your HEALTH

Choosing the Best from
Alternative & Conventional Medicine

EXPERTS TO GUIDE YOU.
RESEARCH TO INFORM YOU.
STORIES TO INSPIRE YOU

ROANNE WEISMAN WITH BRIAN BERMAN, M.D.

Code #0111 • Paperback • $16.95

Available wherever books are sold.
To order direct: Phone 800.441.5569 • Online www.hcibooks.com
Prices do not include shipping and handling. Your response code is BKS.